Wellness
Orgasms

The Fun Way to Live Well and Die
Healthy

The Infidel Secrets to REAL Wellness

Donald B. Ardell PhD
Grant Donovan PhD

Follow Don and Grant on

Facebook or Twitter

Don B. Ardell @Donald_WO
Grant Donovan @Grant_WO

Dedicated to Robert Green Ingersoll (1833 -1899), a pioneer of REAL wellness. *The Great Agnostic's* eloquent lectures and profound writings on matters of reason, exuberance and liberty helped inspire this book. Many of his admirers have called him "the most remarkable American most people never heard of." Our readers will not share in this misfortune.

Warning

Please do not read this book if you are easily offended by public masturbation, same sex marriage, abortion on demand, religious ridicule, free speech or the idea that your life is meaningless and irrelevant.

We wrote this book for those wanting fun lives, so if you prefer orgasms to hell-fires, happiness over fear, love over cruelty and freedom over obedience, this book is for you.

We believe religions are a pox on humanity and a toxin that poisons everything. So, be aware before you begin that we lambast religion mercilessly throughout, with no theocracy-seeking bishop or caliphate-seeking ayatollah spared.

We view REAL wellness, a term you will come to understand, as the antidote to superstition, faith, dogma, subservience and the subjugation of many to ludicrous falsehoods.

This book explores the eclectic secrets of living a life rich in Wellness Orgasms (WOs), so religious zealots, New Age crackpots, cult members, Tea Partiers, spiritualists, Luddites, despots, people who mistreat animals and anyone else predisposed to intolerance and irrationality should be especially careful.

Why? Because we are psychological freedom fighters for joy and personal sovereignty who rather delight in challenging customs, traditions, policies and social norms infected with what we believe are pernicious elements that spread misery and inflict harm.

WOs are about having fun and learning to embrace our inherently meaningless lives with enthusiasm and exuberance. We offer a REAL wellness mindset as an alternative to the prevailing wellness orthodoxy that seeks primarily to avoid disease.

Disease focused groups have hijacked the term *wellness* over recent decades and now it's time to take it back.

There is nothing wrong with the absence of disease or the reduction of high-risk behaviors but neither even remotely resembles REAL wellness. We have no objections to corporate wellness programs trying to cajole fat people into losing weight. We even support drug companies that provide treatments for physical and mental dysfunctions. However, such initiatives should not be associated with any kind of wellness, let alone REAL wellness.

REAL wellness addresses the active and rational pursuit of an orgasmic life filled with positive sensations and the full experience of being alive.

You must never feel guilty for delighting in explosive sensations of unbounded happiness, teary-eyed happiness or even serene contentment. While such sensations may often be transient, they can and should be pursued as part of daily life.

Our purpose in writing this book is to provoke discussion on the advantages of pursuing REAL wellness through scientific reasoning, exuberance, athleticism and the endless pursuit of liberty.

Finally, be warned that the book is just a collection of thoughts based on our extensive reading of the world and while we make reference to the thoughts of many others, you will need to "Google It" if you want verification. It's not our job to do all the work for you, so please don't believe us like we're offering some sort of gospel. Every day's a good day to start thinking critically!

Your Right To Take Offense

The WO philosophy rests on a conscious awareness that modern discoveries about the natural world are vastly superior to the superstitious inanities and insanities of man's ancient past and religious present.

Not that we don't have our heroes from the ancient past. We are fond of several Greek philosophers, particularly Epicurus, who among other profundities observed, no fewer than 23 centuries ago, "there will be nothing to hinder an infinity of worlds."

So it's no surprise to fans of Epicurus that modern astronomers have discovered 370 exoplanets outside our solar system. These reason-guided scientists have demonstrated that our own Milky Way galaxy alone harbors 100 billion stars, billions of which have planetary systems not unlike our own. It's a pity Epicurus is not around to say, "I told you so."

Like Epicurus, we can thrill at the magic of nature. And while the natural world promises us nothing, it doesn't threaten us with eternal misery, either. The universe is infinitely greater and boundlessly more modest than any gods' people have invented to bargain with or worship, kill, sacrifice or die for.

There remains no evidence whatsoever of any transcendent purpose for our being here, so the challenge is to enjoy multiple WOs daily on the short journey to death.

If you're delighted or offended in any way while reading this book, please feel free to share your thoughts. We appreciate all feedback, wherever it falls along the continuum from "You're hell bound" to "Will you marry me?"

If our ideas about the nature of REAL wellness and ways others can benefit from embracing WO thinking lead some to conclude we are guilty of blasphemy, nudity, vegetarianism, irreverence, naturalism, secular humanism or anything else true or false, well, no worries. Always remember, we don't care!

You can catch us on Facebook or Twitter and we will be happy to engage in some meaningless conversation of WO proportions. Friend or foe to our ideas, we welcome your observations, criticisms and suggestions. We also recognize and appreciate your right to say what you think and our right to respond any way we choose.

The WO, REAL Wellness and Meaninglessness

EXPLORING WELLNESS ORGASMS

Remember the orgasm? That feeling of sheer pleasure when all your worries fall away and you are immersed in a most desirable sensation? If you've never had an orgasm without guilt or shame, take it from us; it's a magical experience.

Then again, you may have had similar feelings in other ways, such as when joyfully paralyzed in paroxysms of sidesplitting laughter, the moment of exultation when a feat of personal importance is realized, like crossing the finish line having completed your first marathon, 5K or triathlon, or the joy of surprise reunions with long missed friends and relatives.

Of course, Wellness Orgasms (WOs) can take more modest and more frequent forms, such as appreciating the pleasure of being with or talking to treasured friends, enjoying a delicious meal in a great setting, listening to beautiful music, riding a bike or swimming on a gorgeous morning, singing or dancing to your favorite tune or otherwise immersing yourself in countless situations wherein you have the presence of mind to be aware of your good fortune, the priceless gift of the occasion and the love of someone beside you; all providing a splendid sense of true wellbeing.

Each of these glorious moments can provide true WOs and the more you have during your life, the better your life will be. Perhaps governments should fund a scientific, randomized double blind longitudinal study to help establish minimal daily requirements for WOs.

The U.S. government would probably do so, if not for the fact the Christian Right would throw a Jesus fit. So, being quite fond of pleasure seeking and knowing time is short, we have made it our business to study and embrace WOs as key elements of good health and a REAL wellness lifestyle.

WOs are an important part of effective functioning. They are part of an encompassing world view that can help you stay fit, happy and healthy even when you would otherwise be too tired, stressed, desperate or depressed to really care.

Some people experience multiple WOs on a daily basis, while others struggle to have one a month and even then they feel guilty about it.

WOs are at the center of all good feelings. They are blocked or enhanced by the way you choose to see the world, where you live, who you live with, the conversations you have and the stories you tell yourself.

More specifically, after many decades seeking insights to the critical secrets of a long, happy and healthy life, we find immersion with happy and healthy people to be the number one success factor. That's correct, hanging around with healthy and happy types will make you healthy and happy. It will increase your WO count exponentially.

And given we're all just sitting around waiting to die, why not spend your time enjoying each moment immersed in the thinking and behavioral patterns of the healthiest people you can find. Trust us, it's much better than mixing with depressing religious types or eating fast food with your fat friends.

The company you keep matters more than the food you eat. Successful choices over time of WO-friendly life partners, friends and others are nutrients that can and will sustain your wellbeing as surely as the choices you make around quality foods and worthy exercise habits.

THE POWER OF IMMERSION IN WO CONVERSATIONS

Your conversations shape your thought processes and behaviors.

Every culture, be it family, work, social or societal, is driven in behavior terms by its memes; by its self-replicating thoughts and ideas. If you want to be a criminal, get yourself into prison and do some hardcore associating with real criminals. If you want to be a radical Muslim, join ISIS or the Taliban. But if you want to be happy, healthy and wise then make sure your conversations are with happy, healthy and wise people.

The power of immersing yourself in conversations is so strong that you will quickly become just like the people you regularly converse with. No other conscious effort is required.

Consistent immersion in a pattern of thought, conversation or behavior will produce a sustained personal experience that mirrors the experience of others around you and will rewire your neurological pathways. This will happen regardless if the immersion experience is positive or negative, as we see in the "Stockholm Syndrome."

Put yourself in conversations of a repetitive nature relative to your desires. Don't expect quick results but don't be surprised if you make progress rapidly. In the case of healthy choices, get clear on the nature of such choices. That is, what the results you want really look and feel like.

Talk about the goal with others who enjoy what you want. Break away from the comfortable, the known but possibly ruinous associations that inhibit what you want. The famous architect and suffragist, Florence Luscomb (1887 - 1985), urged as much:

> The tragedy in the lives of most of us is that we go through life walking down a high-walled land with people of our own kind, the same economic situation, the same national background and education and religious outlook. And beyond those walls, all humanity lies, unknown and unseen, and untouched by our restricted and impoverished lives.

Avoid people and environments where conversations undermine what you want. Consider that what you took for granted growing up might be complete nonsense.

The right or functional versus the wrong or disabling conversations for your quality of life are as profound as the difference between day and night, summer and winter, water and fire, and freedom and tyranny.

For example, you may have inhabited a family, cult or community for decades in which the near total, unchallenged reality was Christian fundamentalism. Where, amongst other insufferable nonsense, devotion was accorded to an ancient code of laws and fables judged sacrosanct, infallible and inspired by a bullshit supernatural being. In this case, you would most likely have grown up in a mentally high-walled maximum insecurity zone.

The book to which everyone around you would have bowed is, in reality, the antithesis of what's truly needed to evolve a free life and make exuberant choices, with reason and joy.

Charles Southwell described the Bible quite differently from what you probably accepted growing up, in an apparently normal world that was really full of highly toxic conversations.

> *The Bible has been for ages the idol of all sorts of blockheads, the glory of knaves and the disgust of wise men. It is a history of lust, sodomies, wholesale slaughtering, and horrible depravity; that the vilest parts of all other histories, collected in one monstrous book, could scarcely parallel. The Oracle of Reason via Politics, 1790-1900, Edward Royle, 1976*

As a WO rule, avoid toxic conversations and immerse yourself extensively in conversations with the healthiest people you can find.

WHAT MAKES LIFE WORTH LIVING?

What gives your meaningless life meaning?

Is it the company of and conversations with your partner, parents or children and the sensations associated with such conversations? Is it somehow related to nature? Perhaps it's an experience, such as eating, laughing or certain emotional thrills? Maybe the best of your life comes from achievements or acquisitions? Perhaps from nurturing your artistic or other talents?

More likely it's a combination of some of these and other events, circumstances, experiences and feelings.

What are the highlight elements in your life that have made life worthwhile so far?

Our observations suggest the things that make life worthwhile and cherished are not the watershed moments. They are not your highlights or notable achievements, successes or milestones most likely to turn up in your obituary.

The home run you hit as a kid that won the game and got you carried off the field? It probably won't make the cut. That ceremony and ensuing raucous reception when you married the prettiest girl or the most handsome man on the planet? Nope. How about the arrival of your first born, winning a valuable prize at a game of chance or scoring big time with someone for whom you had lusted for years? Forget about it, events like these are unlikely to have been prime factors in making your life worthwhile.

These kinds of events were epic and triumphant moments at the time but they are too few to sustain wellbeing. No matter how smart, successful, rich, handsome, beautiful, famous or "blessed" you might be, the spectacular and thrilling are too few in number and spaced too far apart to secure an expanding, WO-level of health and happiness.

To attain and sustain wellbeing and make life worth living, in the richest sense of the phrase, you need daily fixes. A life worthwhile and fulfilling is one of daily exuberances of the multiple WO kind based in the activities and conversations with those you really like.

TAKING A RISK FOR WO

WOs are the antidote for lives that are Hobbesian in the sense of being "solitary, poor, nasty, brutish and short," not to mention irrational and thoroughly unwell.

WOs are the opposite of the black holes that lurk in interstellar space, unseen but destructive beyond description. Unlike the black holes scattered throughout the universe, WOs are benevolent. Rather than sucking in and destroying all matter in a vortex of no escape, WO holes make it possible to escape from the surly bonds of dull, unhealthy lives.

One barrier to experiencing regular WOs is the fear of risk taking. But the hesitation to take chances with the unfamiliar or initiatives at odds with what others think are improper, sinful, fattening, immoral, blasphemous or hazardous, must be resisted.

It's natural to fear doing out-of-the-ordinary activities or thinking differently because we are very much constrained by our awareness that some people are easily offended and you can get into trouble trying to innovate or break new ground.

We live in an era of political correctness (PC) where the PC climate puts restrictions on frank discussions. Few want to ruffle tender feelings or be seen as sexist, racist, ageist, atheist or any other "ist" because so many people are quick to take offense at perceived slights, real or more often imagined. As a result, attempts to address the topics that are off limits, to provide a different perspective or to address issues deemed personal or otherwise delicate are usually avoided or quickly shut down by the thought police.

A willingness to break from established norms, to look beyond the mold or otherwise to defy convention of staid traditions is critical for WO development.

To find WOs, search out websites, lectures, conferences and agreeable people that encourage, enable and facilitate a free exchange of ideas. Select a few controversial issues that matter to you and become more comfortable with multiple points of view on topics beyond exercise and fitness, diets and nutrition and all the well-traveled topics of a medical nature.

A PERSONAL PUSH FOR WO

In the spirit of pushing boundaries to see what happens, we delivered a Wellness Orgasm workshop cum seminar at the 1993 National Wellness Conference (NWC) in Stevens Point, Wisconsin.

Note that we have been promoting WOs since the early 1990's, so it's a philosophy with a pedigree.

Anyway, the workshop received sensationally high ratings and much public acclaim. In fact, many still refer to that year's conference as the year of the WO. However, the organizers were well and truly spooked. We have not been allowed since to reprise the WO workshop at the NWC.

In 1993, pre internet porn for the kids, just hearing the word "orgasm" was sufficient to increase heart rates, add stress and bring on a mixture of guilt and scandal. At the conference, you might have thought something wicked, sinful, illegal or inappropriate was taking place. That may sound alluring but all we showed, in a fun way, was how anyone can achieve a state of WO, without removing any clothing or drawing a lot of attention to themselves.

We believe it's healthy and WO-enhancing to do more than simply tolerate speech you don't agree with — we favor encouraging it. Support others to say whatever they like, no matter how dumb, offensive or jejune their benighted opinions might be. Doing so is an effective way to protect and enjoy our own freedom to speak in ways that may upset others.

To promote attendance at the now infamous NWC session, we posted warnings in flyers and on billboards days before the event warding off the easily offended. It simply read:

> Be warned. This is an x-rated workshop, the first ever at the National Wellness Conference. Do not attend if you are easily offended by sacrilege, political incorrectness or heresy in general or flag burning, nudity, pornography or human sacrifices in particular. This workshop is not advised for wellness fundamentalists, morose people attached to 12-step support programs, the devout who want to stay that way, victim-types who think they are terminally dysfunctional, seasoned conference-goers addicted to hugging, spiritual types into hand-holding and guitar music or anyone not willing to take full responsibilities for his/her feelings,

emotions and bladder control. Anyone who likes vegemite, Dan Quayle, the Green Bay Packers or accordions should also stay away. Take a hike around the reservoir or something.

Not surprisingly, the warnings had the intended effect of securing a very large crowd, to the point of over-flowing.

The topics we addressed and the formats we selected for the session were designed to entertain, inform, motivate and arouse; they were also intended to test the limits of free speech. We wanted to lower barriers we thought would inhibit exuberant wellness. We also wanted to introduce new material to the wellness agenda and give participants a chance to be a little outrageous.

In our eyes, we were making a pitch for finding REAL wellness in an unwell world. We championed freedom of thoughts, feelings and actions. Our session was seen, by us at least, as a chance to modestly celebrate uninhibited, spontaneous and frank discussions on whatever topics attendees wanted to address. It was designed to provide psychological liberation from norms that inhibit open discussions. The specific objectives were to identify:

1. Three reasons why it is crucial to position the wellness movement away from the disease model of risk reduction

2. Five ways to expand perspectives regarding what wellness can and should be about

3. Ten principles of freedom vital to every wellness seeker

4.   At least five techniques for shaping a higher order of discussion about serious issues of personal freedom

5.   An alternative way to assess the potentials of "average" citizens to self-manage

The focus of the workshop was not really about orgasms or sex but any topic that attendees might wish to address that could have an impact on wellness lifestyles for themselves and others.

The areas that were specifically mentioned were the pros and cons of drug policies, religion and the institution of marriage. All had a great time, though a tiny handful of the standing-room only crowd expressed displeasure at the frank discussions and other selective elements of the seminar that they found offensive. However, none could claim they were not warned!

The majority gave extremely high marks to the session, noting how much they appreciated the interactive format and groundbreaking nature of the seminar, including audience participation in mini-debates, an opening dance by university students, a WO slide show, several musical pieces, quizzes, skits and simulated performances not seen before or since at the NWC.

It's a pity the session was not videotaped. If it had been, the National Wellness Institute could have made a lot of money, for those in attendance still reminisce about it at reunions these many years later. Come to think of it, we regret not taping it ourselves; we would have made a fiscal killing. Fortunately, we still have rights to the movie!

COULD WOs SAVE THE WORLD?

Lacking medical credentials, we are unable to conduct actual autopsies on deceased, world-class WO paragons to confirm our hypothesis that the power of WOs may very well result from neurological changes in the brain's medial prefrontal cortex.

On the other hand, we have interviewed scores of WO savants, in a dozen countries across the globe and our analysis suggests that WOs are usually associated with lavish mental imagery, multifaceted but wholesome fantasies, increased aptitudes and hallucinogenic synaptic convulsions, all of which seem to trigger unprecedented levels of creative impulses.

Given their exquisite logical nature, we wonder what effects WOs might have had on human history, if only our discoveries had been made much earlier. If so, would humanity be saddled with holy wars between fanatical sects, crusades, inquisitions and persecutions for the past few thousand years?

This is not to suggest that anyone should start a campaign to have us invited to Oslo next year for a Nobel Peace Prize. We're too modest for that sort of thing. We'd be embarrassed.

Still, just think about it. What if WOs had been better understood and cultivated during the Bronze Age? Perhaps the boundlessly cruel tragedies attending the invention of modern religions might well have been entirely avoided.

Humanity needs a global breakthrough of understanding and desire for genuine wellbeing both physical and mental. Advances in human nature away from intolerance and fanaticism, irrationality and superstition are as important to our future happiness as are the arts and sciences. The promotion of WO perspectives might hasten the day when humans are able and willing to focus more on life enhancements and less on the things that make them poor and miserable.

BARRIERS TO WO

Perhaps the most common barrier to the experience of life enriching WOs, in both good and trying times, is mind-emptiness. To be in the WOment is key to seizing the slightest opportunity to turn a thought or experience into a WO. Paradoxically, the best way to master this kind of life-enriching mindfulness is to consciously recognize the pervasive reality of mind-numbing emptiness to which many have become accustomed.

Another barrier is chronic depravity. When you are raised in and otherwise settled into an environment characterized by dogmas and rituals that imprison the brain and corrupt the heart, that produces quiet desperation, fear, dysfunction, boredom, anger and other forms of negativity, you will not be alert to opportunities for having a good WO.

A third barrier is the puritanical hangover, a dark element in the evolutionary process. Wherever you live, your mind has been affected by inherited changes in human populations of an evolutionary nature. Your genetics are subtly different in adaptive ways from even a few generations down your family tree. Successive alterations do not seem to have favored WO skills. Human nature over the last century or so has favored survivor qualities, not the transcendent tendencies of REAL wellness. In some ways, we must overcome our nature to populate our moments WO-fully.

We have touched lightly on the fourth barrier, religion; the worst pox on the earth – ever! Religion promotes the deadly anti-WOs of intolerance, righteousness, cruelty, insularity and closed mind-edness. While reason, liberty, exuberant fun, joy, happiness, laughter, music and dancing are perniciously close to sin, wicked-ness and eternal damnation.

A fifth barrier, poor health, brings pain, diminished energy, the lure of drugs and fear of outcomes fraught with lessened capacity and the possibility of premature death. While only one of these states eliminates future WOs, none facilitates them, either. This barrier, more than most, reinforces the importance of a wellness lifestyle.

A sixth barrier, low self-worth, creates emotional and mental walls around the very idea of making time for WOs. The "I am not worthy" mindset is not nutrient rich soil. It is not the mental en-vironment in which WOs are likely to sprout. Even when, against all odds, a WO-pregnant moment breaks the surface, it is unlikely to be of any real use. The wondrous gift will fade and expire be-fore the unfortunates can recognize and enjoy these life-giving wonders.

A seventh barrier, poverty, colors everything, closes doors and traps the financially afflicted in full-time struggles at the lowest levels in the hierarchy of needs.

CRITICAL WO ENHANCERS

There may be many WO-barriers but there are also some effec-tive WO-enhancers.

One enhancer is a hair-trigger readiness to pounce like a carni-vore, seizing every edible morsel of WOgastic prey. Opportunities abound, if you are ever alert, with an insatiable appetite for even the tiniest garnish of WO-delectability.

A second WO-enhancer is top-of-the-line physical and mental fitness. This acuity gives you a foundation to deal at your best with changing realities and demands. These include aging, adjusting to work and other environmental changes, dealing with sleep interruptions, coping with inevitable losses and setbacks and maintaining a sense of autonomy and self-sufficiency.

A third WO-enhancer is to make wise choices of mates, friends and other associates, not to mention relatives. You start out with relatives that fate chooses for you but no law says you have to associate with all or any of them by the time maturity and changed circumstances deliver the option to fire those not meeting your high standards of healthy connections. It is critical to recruit, test, weed and plant in the characters that play conversational roles in your life. Nurture WO-enhancing individual relationships.

A fourth enhancer is consistent reliance on reason, science and evidence-based thinking. Recognize the reality that there are no divinely ordained ultimate truths. Claims to the contrary by religious interests are, after serious consideration, ignorant in the extreme.

Ultimate truths are rare in the meaningless chaos of life. Science has given contemporary humans an understanding of the natural world that, until recently, was unavailable throughout human history. The young among us are wiser about existential matters and more inclined to be skeptical and to express doubt about dubious and/or ridiculous claims than we ever were. Today's young seem, according to polls, a lot more likely to reject the inanities and insanities that many dutifully adopted and repeated when they were children. There is WO-enhancement power in recognizing this reality.

DEFINING REAL WELLNESS

The term wellness has been hijacked by the medical profession, corporate health promoters, commercial vendors, faith healers and alternative medicine types and is presently used to promote all manner of disease prevention actions where the absence of disease is the ultimate goal.

The term "wellness" was first coined by Halbert L. Dunn to describe a higher state of wellbeing where freedom, joy, exuberance, rational thinking, athleticism and multiple WOs bring a sense of bountiful life to meaningless existence. Dunn and others, ourselves included, associated wellness then with what we call now, REAL wellness.

So don't be fooled. Resigning yourself to a norm of "not being sick" is the equivalent of setting a low bar for your precious wellbeing. It leads to being okay with all manner of dysfunctional states, including being OK about having a body that is overweight and not particularly fit, like nearly everyone else.

Next comes being OK about being depressed, as often as not, being OK about being tired most of the time. Where does it end? Not a good place and, even worse, before you get to a state of serious dysfunction, you will be having a very ordinary life. Bottom line from a REAL wellness perspective: Don't grow accustomed to mediocrity.

The phrase, REAL wellness, was adopted by Don to clearly distinguish between the vibrant energy and rational thinking of people living way beyond the mere disease avoidance levels of the non-sick.

REAL Wellness is not the absence of disease but rather a purposeful striving to live a healthy, fun-filled life that is based on four pillars or foundations for a more challenging, fulfilling and health-ful standard of wellbeing:

R – rational and evidence-based where reliance is on science rather than revealed "truths" based on claims of revelation or authority

E - exuberance and energy to live with a passion and interest about everything, especially arts, sciences, love, learning, happi-ness and joy

A – athletic embrace of both physical activity and healthy foods that science has shown are conducive to exceptional wellbeing

L – liberty and freedom to think, say and do as you like while phys-ically harming no one and to enjoy these opportunities free of guilt and fear

Reason entails skills in effective decision-making. It is thinking and valuing on the basis of evidence and respect for science. It is a learned cognitive process consistent with the famous *baloney detector* criteria made famous by Carl Sagan. It enshrines skepti-cism and doubt, at least until a claim can be supported by the in-dependent verifications of objective parties. Reason can be con-trasted to faith-based thinking, superstition and "truths" founded on non-testable assertions of revelation, miracles or supernatural events.

Exuberance in the REAL wellness context entails devoting equal attention to qualities of mental health and physical wellbeing. This means understanding the nature and approaches to the re-alization of happiness and joy, meaning and purpose, love and passion, fulfillment, awe and wonder; qualities that poets and philosophers throughout the ages have addressed and revered.

Athleticism is the one dimension that was addressed by Don's original wellness model in *High Level Wellness: An Alternative to Doctors, Drugs and Disease, Rodale, 1977*. In the REAL wellness version of the concept, physical fitness, optimal nutrition, sufficient rest and mental toughness are promoted as interconnected disciplines equally crucial to physical excellence. Both exercise and wise food selections are emphasized for health enhancement rather than for disease avoidance benefits. The latter, of course, is a significant side benefit of enjoying positive levels of physical wellbeing.

Liberty is the fourth dimension of REAL wellness. The "L" for liberty is synonymous with freedom, with the two terms being what Ingersoll viewed as "the blossom and fruit of justice, the perfume of mercy, the seed and soil, the air and light, the dew and rain of progress, love and joy." Liberty is a key element in the pursuit of wellbeing. It is vital in the quest for the best life possible in concert with the other REAL wellness dimensions. By developing skills that enhance personal freedoms, citizens can boost their resistance to and protections against theocratic and other non-democratic forces that seek to change the nature of government in dreadful ways. In America today, the wall the Founders erected to keep religion and government separate is under assault. The right to enjoy freedom from religion continues to be eroded by powerful Religious Right leaders on the Supreme Court, in the U.S. Congress and by politician followers and interest groups in every state in the country.

Fortunately, there are many highly effective organizations dedicated to this great challenge including:

- The Freedom from Religion Foundation

- The American Humanist Association

- Council for Secular Humanism

- Americans United for Church and State

EMBRACING MEANINGLESSNESS

The first step on the road to REAL wellness is to give up any thought that your life has been ordained as part of some mysterious grand plan.

WO seekers embrace the knowledge that their life has occurred by pure genetic chance. It was never meant to be, it just happened.

People who experience multiple WOs understand the chance nature of their meaningless existence and the freedom they have to determine their personal path through life without any fear or reference to kings, queens, despots or gods. In the opening words of a masterful speech entitled "Improved Man" (1891), Ingersoll offered this:

> The improved man will be in favor of universal liberty -- that is to say, he will be opposed to all kings and nobles, to all privileged classes. He will give to all others the rights he claims for himself. He will neither bow nor cringe, nor accept bowing and cringing from others. He will be neither master nor slave, neither prince nor peasant -- simply man.
>
> He will be the enemy of all caste, no matter whether its foundation be wealth, title or power, and of him it will be said: 'Blessed is that man who is afraid of no man and of whom no man is afraid.'

Meaninglessness is liberating. It frees us from the stifling need to conform to the drudgery of daily life or the incessant ranting of religious types who believe strict adherence to worshipping invisible gods today will guarantee a heaven-filled life tomorrow. Details of "life" after death in Valhalla or paradise by any name are not available.

WO seekers embrace meaninglessness because it eliminates the need to achieve, follow deities, worry about mistakes, care what others think and generally be stressed by daily living. No need, either, to give any part of what you earn to support imam or priest, ayatollah, dali lama or pope.

Embracing meaninglessness builds a welcome sense that anything is possible but little is critical. It brings to ever-conscious awareness that life is a short journey, where choice over what you think is the greatest health enhancer, even if you were born, by chance, into a negative social or physical environment.

So our advice is to stop worrying. You are here by chance and you can either bow and cringe to zealots, who want to shape and manage your thoughts, or you can choose the path of WO, where meaninglessness will set you free.

Reason

No amount of belief makes something a fact. James Randi

THINKING RATIONALLY

One way to help master the Zen of meaninglessness is to learn critical thinking. You don't have to be a scientist to appreciate the scientific method and to utilize its basic framework for effective decision-making. Decide matters large and small based on facts, observation, investigation, experiments, experience and demonstrations. Consider one of Ingersoll's seven qualities of "Improved Man":

> *The Improved Man will be self-poised, independent, candid and free. He will be a scientist. He will observe, investigate, experiment and demonstrate. He will use his sense and his senses. He will keep his mind open as the day to the hints and suggestions of nature. He will always be a student, a learner and*

*a listener - a believer in intellectual hospitality. In
the world of his brain there will be continuous summer, perpetual seedtime and harvest. Facts will be
the foundation of his faith. In one hand he will carry
the torch of truth and with the other raise the fallen.*

It is an unbelievably WO-filled experience to sort fact from nonsense. It's such a powerful feeling to be armed with information
that can help you make better life decisions. The alternative is
pitiful, wretched and wildly popular reliance on prayers and sup-
plications, fastings and genuflections, superstition and the hear-
say of the ill informed.

Rational thought builds justifiable confidence and enhances
your sense of wonder. It helps you explore fascinating facts
about how the universe was formed, why the sun is critical for
human life and how your blood delivers food and oxygen to the
100 trillion cells in your body. None of this can be found in holy
books.

Cars cannot move, planes cannot fly and cancers cannot be cured
by prayer.

Critical thinking skills can also help you choose REAL wellness behaviors over pernicious and ill-considered actions that can bring
personal harm, to sort fact from fiction in advertising, to see
through political spin, to fight back against religious nonsense and
to avoid unscrupulous bankers and lovers.

Using reason by thinking rationally is the first and most critical
skill of REAL wellness but, like any skill, it takes time and effort
to develop. Many people are not inclined toward reason-based
thinking because social immersion makes it easier to go along
with customs, traditions, rituals and practices that were part of

growing up and fitting in with everyone else. Reason takes more energy than watching drivel on television, spreading gossip on social media and letting other people tell you what to think, buy and feel.

The reality when it comes to rational scientific thinking is that most people Cantdoit because they lack the training and discipline required.

The greater danger with going brain dead is losing the ability to recognize the circus-like forms of nonsense that pass for normal and decent. Think of the multi-millionaire TV preachers, with mega-churches seeking more and more donations. The pedophile priests undetected for years by gullible true believers and all the abuses of religions infringing on public policy under the guise of religious freedoms.

Ultimately it may not matter what you think in a meaningless world but, while you're here, critical thinking builds wisdom and wonderment of epic WO proportions, while blind faith harms the innocent and leads to holy horrors without end.

THE STORY OF GODS

God does exist in our minds and she is always open for a conversation but let's take a rational look at whether gods exist in fact?

Throughout the 200 thousand-plus years of human history, many thousands of gods have been worshipped in all regions of the world. So the worshipping of unsighted gods is a proven fact. Yet, no evidence is available to indicate, let alone prove, that these perceived gods are any more than the figment of desperate imaginations.

Even if gods do not exist, as we maintain, one question is often asked: Does true god belief or fake belief, for that matter, have WO-like benefits? Does belief provide some measure of health-enhancing certainty that many people crave? Does it deliver a positive mental state?

The answer for some people is clearly yes. The belief in the supernatural provides some with a serene confidence that has WO outcomes. For others, the story is different because their god is a tyrant who rules by the fear of hell.

Atheists are free of such fears and experience an independence of thought that adds substantially to their sense of wellness. They are free to follow their own ethical, reasoned and compassionate thoughts without the fear of heavenly retribution.

Atheism, free-thought, agnosticism, secular humanism and just being an infidel leads to strong self-confidence and a level of self-reliance that is actualizing beyond any level of the Maslow hierarchy. The WO value of atheism is never mentioned in corporate or other wellness programming. Raising the topic would so upset the religious types that the resulting controversy would end the wellness program. Religionists are not trained to be open to ideas at odds with their respective faiths.

Gods exist in modern times because parents, relatives and adults in religious schools pass along such beliefs. The timing of this transmission is critical because the religionists know that this is the period when the child's brain is malleable and the child is most easily led. The only hope for the child is exposure to other perspectives, support for doubt and for scientific thinking. The next step for liberation from superstition is exposure to WO supportive communities.

It's a big ask to expect parents raised in religious immersion to be comfortable allowing a child to access rational thinking skills early in life, even if granting such freedoms enables the child to make better personal decisions around everything from peer selection to drug use.

THE WAR ON DRUGS

Are illicit drugs bad or is the war on drugs a desperate bid by god-fearing control freaks to make everyone behave? Is it more about mass human behavior control than the damage illicit drugs might do? Is it more about a misguided drive for perfect people when the real need may be for mind altering drugs to block out the imperfections?

Do the facts support a police state war on drugs or are there other, more WO-enhancing ways to manage the perceived problem in a meaningless world?

So many questions for future discussion but right now we know America has spent well over one trillion dollars and made more than 50 million arrests in the 40-plus years since the war on drugs began, with no end in sight. Is the country better off now than when the war began? Is there less drug use?

Do the results suggest we should fight the battle for another 40 years, if necessary, until we get the users and abusers to surrender unconditionally? Is it worth another five or 10 trillion dollars and 50 million more arrests? Will we be better off then?

We're skeptical and we're also big on liberty. Big on the freedom for people to make their own, informed choices without government control. The lack of freedom to make personal decisions is WO-debilitating.

We are skeptical about the drug war, in good measure because we value liberties and the rights of individuals to make self managed decisions as critical prerequisites for WOs. We would be against the drug war even if we were winning it on the cheap, which clearly we're not.

The drug war has created a totalitarian system that produces crime and criminals, fills jails, prisons and cemeteries; it also destroys the prospects of large segments of the underclass. It is completely at odds with personal freedoms. It is paternalistic and oppressive. Its unintended consequences are destructive beyond belief.

If there is an antonym for WO, it's WID - *worseness impotent dysfunction*. The lamentable war has unleashed a maelstrom of WID's that have caused America, Mexico and other nations around the globe to become poorer, meaner and more dangerous.

America and other states need a serious rethink because war on the production, distribution and use of marijuana, cocaine, heroin and other more or less universally illegal chemicals has hidden the grief associated with legal drugs. Over-the-counter and prescription drugs kill some 15,000 Americans annually just from overdoses.

Opioid painkillers are a $9 billion annual business. They are highly addictive and they cause brain modifications, not for the better. These legal drugs reduce any chance users have to experience WOs because they damage the brain's pleasure centers. With regular use, the brain needs more of the drug just to feel normal, so REAL wellness becomes unattainable to people hooked on either medically prescribed or illegal drugs.

More deaths are attributed to overdoses of prescription medications than from heroin, cocaine and all other illegal drugs combined. Opioid abuse is a key element in the fact that drug overdoses count as the single largest cause of accidental death in America, a higher toll than traffic accidents.

The irrational, unthinking use of illicit and legal chemicals is the problem, not the drugs themselves. So, again, what we need to solve the drug problem is better thinking skills, less control and command, more education, more compassion, less punishment and the elimination of degradation and revenge.

We believe no drugs of any kind should be illegal to use. Production should be managed only by regulatory agencies.

Free distribution to addicts and others who want to ruin themselves should be the only policy. By giving the stuff away, there will be no underground markets supporting the treacherous, violent and catastrophic enterprises that grow, cultivate, smuggle and kill to defend their turfs.

Yes, there may be more drug users cultivated by free distribution and more mental and physical health problems for the medical system to manage but it matters not how people choose to kill themselves; that is their free choice. What matters is the redirection of trillions to the compassionate care and end state support for people not finding WOs in their accidental world experience.

The majority of the world's populations are born into struggling financial circumstances, with limited opportunity, so mind altering drugs offer some real comfort to their un-chosen, random and meaningless existence. But even rich lawyers and stock traders, who finds it all a bit tedious, need their mind-altering substances.

THE WO-FILLED FACTS ABOUT MONEY AND STATUS

So, what is the relationship between your monetary position, your perceived status in society and your likelihood of experiencing multiple WOs throughout your life?

Can more money make you healthier and happier and give you greater access to WOs?

The answer is a big YES!

Modern psychology research, probing the health disparities between rich and poor, suggests your health status is not simply a matter of unequal access to health care but, rather, unequal access to money. We know this because real health disparities exist even in countries where everyone has universal access to free medical treatment.

Norman B. Anderson, a professor at the Harvard School of Public Health, has conducted research on the link between health and money. His research shows that Americans who earn $500,000 a year enjoy fewer health problems and live longer than those making a more than respectable $100,000 per year.

This finding is supported by broader epidemiological studies that suggest a close relationship exists between income, education and occupation on the one hand and health outcomes on the other. A decade-long Whitehall study of 17,350 British civil servants found the relative risk of illness and death increased significantly as a person's job level and financial reward decreased.

The message for those living in the first world is simple: The lower your social status and the less money you have, the greater your risk of both physical and psychological health problems.

Put simply, for most people it seems that less money means fewer WOs. Sad but mostly true.

It's also true that people at the lower end of the socioeconomic spectrum tend to smoke more, eat worse and live in unhealthier environments. They also have lower levels of education, fewer social skills and grim prospects for much that is good and life enhancing.

Insufficient wealth is an under-appreciated health hazard and one of the highest obstacles imaginable to a WO-filled life.

Money may not guarantee happiness but it provides a doorway to options that people without money cannot access.

Lack of money and status is a major cause of illness and death. People without either, in a meaningless and chance-based world, lead WO-less lives and die earlier than people with money and status, even if they can, against all odds, follow sound diet, exercise and other lifestyle patterns.

It seems low socioeconomic status directly impairs the immune system's ability to ward off infections. Those on the lowest status rungs are at the highest risk of developing infections; the unemployed and under employed are four and a half times more likely to get sick when exposed to the cold virus than people with jobs and money.

THE RICH AND THE WO

America's richest one percent control more wealth than the poorest 40%.

Income inequality has been a long-term problem and the gap continues to increase, so it's possible but unlikely that you will ever work your way into the top one percent wealth-wise. Some exceptional good fortune might get you there but, if you are not already there, don't let your happiness depend on it.

The economic disparity is challenging because the one to 40 percent divide is the mother of all divides. This matters in a WO sense because such disparities create unhealthy living environments.

The International Monetary Fund (IMF) recently addressed wealth disparities in a report to all 188 member nations. Along with a wide range of economists, policy leaders, social trend experts and a range of public and private organizations, the IMF forecasts the great income inequality chasm will slow economic growth and risk social upheavals, if not revolutions, as the divide inevitably grows ever larger.

What might be done in the US to spread the wealth without inhibiting growth?

Here are a few suggestions, though some might be precisely the kind of reforms that would be used to inflame Tea Party types to demand secession.

- Raise income and property taxes at the higher levels far more progressively than is now the case. How high? How about setting the tax rate for all income over $10 million annually at 90 percent? Okay, what about 75 percent or raising the level for such redistribution to annual incomes over $20 million? The Koch Brothers would still have plenty left over to support Right Wing candidates for Congress and state legislatures. Who can't live quite well on that kind of bounty? Such changes will enable tens of millions of poor and middle income Americans to enjoy greater prosperity, with enhanced funding for our environments, for social welfare, health, education and the infrastructure required for every community to function well. Such fiscal policies might even lead to lower dysfunctions (e.g., crime rates, bankruptcies) and increase peace and serenity levels.

- Limit the amount of wealth that can be transferred to heirs. Nothing too revolutionary, maybe only $50 million from all sources could be passed along using estate tax policies. Alright, how about $100 million? Couldn't any kid live on that?

- Eliminate sales taxes on all but extreme luxury goods. Start with goods that even Republicans would struggle to claim are not truly luxury items, such as private jets, homes over $2 million dollars, autos over $100 grand and so on. Make the sales tax at least 25 cents on the luxury dollar.

- Eliminate mortgage interest rate tax deductions on loans of $1 million or more. Present tax policies allow unlimited interest rate deductions. In effect, this means everyone supports the extravagant leverage of wealth by the super-rich.

- Dramatically curtail the wealth-sheltering practice of setting up foundations. Causes deemed worthy would become public policy choices. At present, charities are set up, funded and controlled by the rich and powerful for the rich and powerful and the causes they favor.

- Eliminate tax concessions for religions.

Whew. That should be a sufficient starter set of modest reforms. As Robert Green Ingersoll extolled in 1890:

The Improved Man will not give his life to the accumulation of wealth. He will find no happiness in exciting the envy of his neighbors. He will not care to live in a palace while others who are good, industrious and kind are compelled to huddle in huts and dens. He will know that great wealth is a great burden, and that to accumulate beyond the actual needs of a reasonable human being is to increase not wealth but responsibility and trouble.

THE HEALTH DIVIDE

Americans may take their religion on faith because it's inculcated over two decades of formative programming, with little or no exposure to alternative explanations of reality.

Recent research, however, suggests that few sentient beings are so easily fooled when it comes to the wealth divide, with a Pew Research Center Survey showing more than half (61%) the US population believes the economic system favors the wealthy, which of course it does, overwhelmingly.

The population is less enlightened, however, with respect to the lifestyle and wellbeing divide. This is true despite the fact the gap, between the tiny fraction of Americans immersed in elevated states of sound physical and mental functioning and nearly everyone else, is much greater than the income divide.

Most overweight, stressed, unhappy, unfit, mentally suspect folk, in unsatisfying work situations, who lack passions and skills for advancing positive, life-affirming goals may feel they're doing okay. Of course, this cannot be true or the US would not need a

$3 trillion health care or, more accurately, chronic illness-focused medical system.

So, can REAL wellness be rendered more appealing to the indifferent, essentially ineligible masses? Can this happen to the point that everyone will commit to transforming their daily thinking and behavioral patterns into glorious lifestyles consistent with their personal potentials and possibilities?

The short answer is no; 70 to 90 percent of the population are not even close to a function consistent with REAL wellness and are never going to get there. For example, people who are not happy in their work, are not fit for it, do too much of it and have a scarce sense of success in it are unlikely to experience much change over their lifetime.

Yet, when all is said and done, there is still a glimmer of hope for anyone who wants to make the effort because, even with a moderate effort, someone disadvantaged in dozens of ways has a better shot at REAL wellness than they have of ever breaking into the ranks of the super duper, wealthy one percent.

And the really good news is that REAL wellness without wealth is better than wealth without a REAL wellness.

EXPLORING THE WO-DEBILITATING POVERTY TRAP FURTHER: INCARCERATION

We know that poverty leads directly to sickness but while low social status is WO-debilitating, poverty is WO-eliminating.

In economic terms, the Poverty Trap is a self-perpetuating condition. Just as an economy caught in a downward cycle suffers from persistent underdevelopment, so too does the Poverty Trap create a vicious, self-perpetuating spiral into despair, desperation and destructive personal behaviors. Those caught in the cycle have little chance of ever experiencing even simple WOs.

The Poverty Trap in America is a matter of public policy and corporate greed. The top one percent of income earners do all they can to protect their 90 percent share of all the accumulated wealth. Among the strategies they favor are higher rates of incarceration of the less wealthy. Naturally, this only serves to increases the economic, social and health divides.

The US now imprisons more people in absolute numbers and per capita than any other country on earth. With five percent of the world population, the U.S. hosts upward of 20 percent of its prisoners. About 2 million Americans currently live behind bars and many millions more are on parole or probation. Many are there for minor crimes or small time drug use.

Sociologists Bruce Western from Harvard and Becky Pettit from the University of Washington have shown how poverty creates prisoners and how prisons fuel poverty. Their research concludes that once a person has been incarcerated, his or her earning power is significantly reduced and their ability to climb out of poverty, even decades after release, is limited at best.

A more damning fact is that in 1980, 10 percent of black high-school dropouts were incarcerated. By 2008, that number was 37 percent. As the song goes, this bad moon is on the rise.

The scale of black incarceration is staggering. When researchers factor prisoners into government unemployment numbers, the statistics show that fewer than 30 percent of black male high school dropouts are currently employed. Imagine, 70 percent of these unskilled young are jobless with few prospects.

Such unemployment figures are usually associated with failed Third World states rather than one of the wealthiest economies on earth. It augurs ill for personal WO opportunities and long-term social stability.

And getting out of prison doesn't bring much relief from despair for those in the society who are most disenfranchised. One study found that after being out of prison for 20 years, more than three-quarters of ex-cons, who did not finish high school, were below the bottom 20 percent of income earners. Even worse, children of prisoners are more likely to live in poverty, to end up on welfare and to suffer the sorts of serious emotional problems that make holding jobs more difficult.

Exuberance

BORN TO DIE

To be born is a bit like receiving a double verdict from a jury despite having done nothing to deserve it. The double verdict: a life sentence and a sentence of death.

With the life sentence, you receive an opportunity, for varying time periods, to dwell with a consciousness and a body under sun and stars. If favored by random good fortune in the lotteries of family, place, genetics and other variables that affect the extent and quality of love, happiness, freedom, knowledge, joy and the wonder you experience, you could be in for a glorious ride lasting many decades. If not so favored, your experiences may be grim.

Your fate could be unbroken hunger and privation, pain and rejection, slavery and unmitigated misery. There is no rhyme or reason that can explain why some infants are born into lives of health and advantage, with prospects for longevity and prosperity, while others are born into squalor and sickness, want, ignorance and grief.

Of course, religionists tell believers that it's all part of a grand plan by one god or another and we're not smart enough to know how they came up with such a plan or whether an environmental impact study was ever done.

As Ingersoll noted in the speech in the Congressional Cemetery in Washington, DC on January 12, 1882:

> *Every cradle asks us whence, every coffin wither. The poor barbarian weeping above his dead can answer the question as substantially and as satisfactorily as the robed priest of the most authentic creed. The tearful ignorance of the one is as consoling as the learned and unmeaning words of the other.*

But, it is just a ride, whether rich and loved, poor and ignored or something in between, the ride of life does not last long, you don't get to go around again and there are no second chances, even if really bad things happen along the way.

These factors are as capricious as they are significant. You get few to no choices, particularly in the first decade or so. It all just happens, like the Big Bang.

Don't take it personally. This is how things are, for you, your linear ancestors, and everyone else. You are born to die but that does not mean you cannot embrace life with all the exuberance you can muster.

That's the REAL wellness challenge.

THE WAITING ROOM

You might think of all of us as gathered in one large waiting room, moving around, reading, watching TV, trying to stay busy, looking to be entertained while we wait to die. Okay, so not a very cheery thought but, nonetheless, a true thought that is liberating if we choose action over sedation and self-reliance over compliance.

Most people do not like thinking about dying, so we look for diversions; busy stuff that helps us feel worthwhile and keeps our mind off our looming demise. It's the penalty for evolving a conscious mind that struggles for meaning in a life without reason, save for any we invent.

Billions embrace gods to help them through while others soldier on regardless.

On what basis do the god believers believe? Well, it would be nice if it were something more but, unfortunately, it's just mind numbing faith.

"Faith," as Mark Twain famously noted, "is believen what you know ain't so."

Faith has been explained as an illogical belief in the occurrence of the improbable.

Despite our intelligence, we embrace folly, a fact not lost on countless observers, including Aldous Huxley:

> *You never see animals going through the absurd*
> *and often horrible fooleries of magic and religion...*
> *Asses do not bray a liturgy to cloudless skies. Nor*
> *do cats attempt, by abstinence from cat's meat, to*

wheedle the feline spirits into benevolence. Only man behaves with such gratuitous folly. It is the price he has to pay for being intelligent but not, as yet, quite intelligent enough.

Of course, much of the busy stuff represents eking out a way to survive and pass on our DNA to the next hapless group, who pass their DNA to the next group and so it goes, forevermore until who knows what?

We try to give our existence meaning when no meaning exists. We arrive on the earth by chance, into unchosen environments, with no pre-determined purpose, do what we're told and sit in the Waiting Room for our time to leave. All our personal achievements provide momentary pleasure but they are meaningless in the bigger, cosmic sense.

THE GOOD NEWS

So, here's the good news from a WO perspective. Once we get through all the thought stages of death and dying, we can start living on our own terms, enjoying our momentary existence and refusing to take orders from the guards in the Waiting Room. Paraphrasing Michel Onfray's *Atheist Manifesto*, some of us prefer philosophers and irreverent comics, radicals, cynics, hedonists, sensualists, scientists and voluptuaries to bishops, popes, rabbis, imams, ayatollahs and mullahs.

Why be cloistered in thought or action by other people who want to control your meaningless existence? Why accept their rules, if you can create your own without infringing on the rights of others?

Play your own game!

It's time to ignore the forces of bureaucracy, politics, marketing and religion and do what makes you happy, enthusiastic and exuberant; provided it's legal, considerate and does not interfere with the happiness of neighbors. As Ingersoll put it:

> *Everyone should be as happy as he can be, provided he is not happy at the expense of another, and no person rightly constituted can be happy at the expense of another.*

The certainty of death and the meaninglessness of life invite us to freely engage in WOs joyfully pursued.

It's time to cheer in the Waiting Room, blissfully aware but not controlled or inhibited by friends, family, teachers, lawmakers, parsons, priests or gods.

That's the beauty of randomly occurring life; you can wait quietly or make a fuss. Either way, best to do it on your own terms, without kowtowing to those who want to control your every thought and action.

Andy Rooney put it this way:

> *We all ought to understand we're on our own. Believing in Santa Claus doesn't do kids any harm for a few years but it isn't smart for them to continue waiting all their lives for him to come down the chimney with something wonderful. Santa Claus and God are cousins.*

CANTDOIT

Right about now you might be questioning the point of it all. That is to say, if there is no meaning and we are just waiting around to die then what is there to live for?

Not everyone can deal with the reality of meaningless, most people Cantdoit; that is, most cannot sustain a REAL wellness-based life in the face of their own mortality.

They struggle to find the desire to question everything, embrace reality, champion liberty and engage athletically in life, with exuberant curiosity. They find it difficult to live a WO existence and inevitably collapse into the mire of obedience, sloth and medical malaise.

Those reared to not question religions will denounce WOs as the hedonistic babble of lost souls but that is because they are ubiquitously surrounded and conditioned by societies largely based on nonsensical world-views, customs and rules.

They are not bad people, just hapless victims of mental evolution steeped in superstition.

Better their atoms formed rocks than flesh but, alas, they are trapped. Searching for comfort in all the wrong places and immersed in a narrative that only the WO-minded can escape.

Imagine a scene similar to that befalling Dorothy in "The Wizard of Oz." While you may start from Kansas, your destination is not Oz.

You are transplanted into the life of a very young person, a female, in a Middle Eastern theocracy governed by warlords, royalty or religious authorities. You are in a Bronze Age culture, even though it's the 21st century. You realize that the beliefs that govern how you live in every imaginable way are extraordinarily constricting and, from your point of view, totally whacky, if not bloody insane. You have the knowledge and aspirations you possess today but in this new situation no opportunities or resources to change your life, even though you desperately wanted to.

Would WOs be difficult to achieve in such a time and place? What would you do, trapped in a culture where you want to change but the environment means you just Cantdoit. What would be the reality of your short and meaningless life?

That's basically how it is where you live now. The difference being in your real world is that the constricting realities around you are harder to recognize and thus, powerfully effective in keeping you stuck. When the conversations are limited, there's nothing keeping you from adopting and even reinforcing the mind-bending nonsense of religious dogmas and all forms of learned stupidity that clogs mental arteries and prevents frequent WOs.

So, can we achieve happiness in a meaningless world?

If our presence on earth is random and our fate equally so, can we find or create paths to exuberance, joy and optimism or are we inexorably destined for a herd-like life, filled with senseless drama, stress, depression, misery and doom?

The answer is "yes we can" for WO seekers (though it won't be easy) but, for the rest, the reality is almost surely "probably not."

THE WAY TO WOs

The first step to exuberant WOs is, to paraphrase Gertrude Stein, accept the fact that there's "no there in the hereafter." This is it; so don't squander the improbable but potentially wondrous opportunities that life offers.

Meaninglessness is great news because we're on our own. We're free to play the game of life and win with a stoic embrace of reason, exuberance, athleticism and liberty.

Here are a few WO tips to help you along your way.

- Commit to having fun by rejecting nonsense and happiness-limiting rules

- Lighten up and take life a little less seriously

- Accept no rule that says you have to believe what others in your clan, culture or organization believes if the doctrine makes no sense

- Recognize that few investments will provide a better return than the time and energy invested thinking for yourself, relying on evidence while guided by tools of reason and science

- Develop a clear sense for what it means to be physically and mentally healthy far beyond the illness avoidance parameters of the medical system

- Engage life with exuberant energy

- Seek serenity in the sounds of your own thoughts and your ability to deflect the babbling noise of others

WHATEVER HAPPENED TO PEACE AND QUIET?

The volume of sound from countless sources has been rising for years. For those whose work or life situations put them in the thick of unnerving sound levels, the hubbub and clamor has become WO-debilitating.

Screaming children on airplanes, general noise from cars, planes, bikes, buses, lawn mowers, garden blowers, TV's, radios, stereos, flatulence and an endless array of other sources seem to fill the air almost incessantly. This can build to stress beyond the pale for some, including a few who might lose control and figuratively or otherwise try to shoot their way out of their misery.

Noise also takes the form of subtle, incessant sound demands competing for your attention; 24-hour news cycles, ads, signs, billboards, emails, social media and nonsense-producing devices that fill time and space.

Given the din, your brain needs access to an easy-to-find, semi-automatic off switch.

You need to create brain cues that are the equivalent of a reverse motion-sensing light switch that can dim unwanted noise levels and protect your brain from an evil menace that threatens WO-serenity levels.

A cacophony of noise does not contribute to wellbeing. Beauty is silent; we have never heard a sunset, a rose or a painting.

Noise dampens exuberance.

Noisome sounds at elevated levels subdue reflections, pensiveness and nuance. Over time, one can suffer a coarsening of mental acuity. Arthur Schopenhauer (1788-1860) understood the problem.

> *Noise is the most impertinent of all forms of inter-*
> *ruption. It is not only an interruption but is also a*
> *disruption of thought.*

He knew a long time ago that noise is extremely WO-debilitating.

The general buzz, jangle and uproar we endure in daily life has consequences, including a lowering of the bar for political fig- ures, who compete for our attention through a tangle of noise. The messages they send assume the masses have hair-trigger at- tention spans, so the messages they convey are quick, loud, dumb and crude. Thus, public figures resort to sound bites and slogans, 147 maximum character tweets and disparaging one-minute at- tack ads.

A numb public today is nearly incapable of holding still for more than ten minutes. Noise has dulled the discipline, the senses and the attention spans of contemporary audiences. Deep, explorato- ry conversation has been lost to a cacophony of chatter.

Amplification is a key element of this WO-inhibiting, health threatening hazard. The risks derive not only from decibels but also from the sheer volume of moronic messaging. We are awash in devices; their misuse and abuse raise crowd sounds to ungodly levels. Visit any public space and you're likely to be distracted by screaming children, emergency vehicle sirens or countless hard-of-hearing cell phone users sprouting nonsense to invisible but equally hard-of-hearing receivers.

Ingersoll once addressed a crowd of 50,000, with not so much as a bullhorn, let alone amplification with sound systems we take for granted. No wonder Eugene Debs called him the "Shakespeare of oratory" and Mark Twain was moved to say, "What an organ is human speech when it is employed by a master."

But, would Ingersoll be heard at all today, even if he could enjoy our beyond-belief technologies? Though he was a hero to James Garfield, Walt Whitman, Ulysses Grant, Margaret Sanger, Andrew Carnegie, Thomas Edison, Henry Ward Beecher and Elizabeth Cady Stanton, among others, his great voice would be muted and lost in the current din.

Research suggests that regular exposure to sounds at 30 decibels and up is associated with high blood pressure, anxiety and stress.

A 2011 report by the World Health Organization and the European Commission's Joint Research Center concluded, after a meta-analysis of epidemiological studies, that repeated exposure to noise pollution may lead to higher blood pressure and fatal heart attacks. The report also confirmed suspicions that chronic noise impairs a child's development, with possible life-long effects on educational attainment and overall health.

Environmental psychologist Arline Bronzaft, from the City University of New York, researched the impact of train noise on child development in the 1970s. She found that reading scores of sixth-grade students in classrooms facing passing trains were a year behind those on the quieter side of the building. Full details are reported in her book "Why Noise Matters" (2011).

Trains aren't the only noise culprits. Children living close to aircraft noise also suffer poor classroom performance. A Munich airport study led by psychologists Staffan Hygge, Gary W. Evans and Monika Bullinger tested the reading, memory, attention and hearing skills of third and fourth grade students living and/or attending school near airport sites. One airport was being phased out as a new facility was being opened in another area of the city. The reading comprehension skills and the long-term memories of children near the closing airport improved once air traffic was rerouted to the new airport, while the performance of children near the new airport declined.

The researchers also found the Munich students near the working airports had significantly higher levels of the stress hormones adrenaline and cortisol. In addition, the students had markedly higher blood pressure readings than children in quieter neighborhoods.

In short, the studies showed that higher levels of noise exposure increased the risks of life-threatening adult illnesses, including high blood pressure, elevated cholesterol and heart disease.

We all know intuitively that sustained exposure to physical noise, the wall of visual messages and our own internal chatter undermine and obstruct WO opportunities. It is time to recognize and promote the value of designing more silence in our lives. It's good for our health and it's great for our WOs.

Various researchers and writers suggest that the conscious practice of silence has many benefits, among them lower stress levels, enhanced happiness and improved brain chemistry. Reduced to the basics, lower sounds levels will help you look and feel younger and enjoy more exuberance.

Silence is WO-filled because it welcomes and is conducive to contemplation and reflection, the exploration of ideas and nuance, occasions critical thought and helps build an intrinsic understanding of life in all its meaningless glory.

Athleticism

GET MOVING

Does it matter if you're fit and healthy in a world without meaning? If we're all doomed to become dust sooner or later, is exercise really worth the bother?

Furthermore, when the evidence around us indicates that most Cantdoit anyway, why struggle? Isn't it better not to have tried than to have labored mightily, day after day, for weeks or perhaps months, eventually giving it up and then feeling dispirited and defeated?

Well, that's for you to decide but we don't recommend resignation. We don't favor low expectations, either, or the helplessness that comes with a fear of failure. We're against all such attitudes for one simple reason; these perspectives are incompatible with WOs.

We personally know that many WOs come from being physically active, eating well and facing meaninglessness with exuberance.

From our perspective, REAL Wellness means, in part, being dramatically fitter than most people your own age, give or take about five years, exercising regularly and dining most of the time on plant-based whole-foods and other comestibles low in animal proteins, sodium, fat and sugar.

It also means exercising on a near-daily basis and refraining from overindulging in alcohol, drugs, all night parties and rock and roll.

Ok, rock and roll and late night parties are fine if they get you dancing and moving but maybe not every night and not if they leave you in a drunken mess.

The real WO challenge is to move often and vigorously.

EXERCISE AND FITNESS: FUNDAMENTALS FOR REAL WELLNESS

Thousands of books can be found in libraries and bookshelves the world over on topics related to exercise and fitness. While most are loaded with worthy content, many do go on beyond a level required to strike at the heart of the matter.

The essentials of exercise and fitness are quite simple.

- Choose physical activities you enjoy sufficiently to perform daily, for an hour or more

- Immerse yourself with others who share your enthusiasm for the chosen physical activity. Affiliating with those like-minded about exercise increases your staying power

- Recognize that exercise should be long enough, hard enough and done often enough to make a difference to your fitness level over time

- Technique matters because form enhances function and adds satisfaction while boosting performance. If you choose swimming for fitness you are far more likely to persevere if you have good stroke, breathing and streamlining skills

- Exercise for health, fun and WO-enhancement. It's too important to pursue for weight loss, medical benefits or problem alleviation, even though such ancillary gains are highly worthwhile

- Take care that you get sufficient rest and adequate sleep. Harvard Medical School research suggests about three-quarters of the U.S. population has intermittent sleep difficulties, worsened, no doubt, by sedentary living. Current scientific consensus suggests most people need a minimum of seven hours of sleep nightly

Pay attention to the most important body organ that affects the quality of your exercise routine; the brain.

Work to develop the neural control center for all that you contemplate and do, including looking after the rest of your body with regular, sufficient exercise. Look for ways to train your brain that will improve its capacity to transmit signals that are positive and encouraging, upbeat, optimistic and guided by reason and common sense.

In the words of George Bernard Shaw:

No diet will remove all the fat from your body because the brain is entirely fat. Without a brain you might look good but all you could do is run for public office.

CHASING SEX

Swimming, biking, running, weight training and other forms of strenuous exertion facilitate and enhance sexual pleasures. Such exercise is consistent with and supports WO-enhancing pursuits of a REAL wellness nature. Yet, sex by itself, without elaborate or devotional preparations, is still quite healthful and delightful.

Naturally, sex works best when done in ways that are safe and consensual and when religious toxins, like guilt and medieval mores are absent from the proceedings.

The promotion of chastity and abstinence is WO-debilitating and stupid to boot. As Aldous Huxley once noted, "Chastity is the most unnatural of the sexual perversions," while Dick Cavett opines, "Abstinence education is surely the worst idea since chocolate-covered ants."

Sex is fun and totally WO-enhancing. Most experts and others who study human sexual activity believe copious sexual activity, with a loving partner or, if you don't have a single caring partner, with loving, trustworthy others, provides generous physical and mental health benefits.

Sex and intimacy boost self-esteem and happiness. *Happiness*, as Ingersoll noted,

Is the only good and everything that adds to the happiness of sentient beings is good and to do the things, and no other that add to the happiness of man is to practice the highest possible religion.

Sex also boosts your immune system. Studies suggest college students who have sex one or more times per week have higher levels of the immunoglobulin A (IgA) antibody than their less *succsexful* peers.

While sex is complicated enough in its own right, religious dogmas have suppressed the dissemination of sexual knowledge to hundreds of millions. This has created all manner of misunderstandings about a fundamental reality for all life forms. In the U.S. and elsewhere, "abstinence education" is a code phrase for the suppression of knowledge.

Here are a few basics every young person should learn as thoroughly as anything else taught in the primary grades. Such knowledge would enable children to better care for their bodies, make more responsible choices and develop more confidence and self-respect.

- Sexual and reproductive anatomy
- Gender identity and orientation be it heterosexual, bisexual, homosexual, transsexual or any other sexual
- Ways in which morals, family, friends, religion, age, life goals and other factors shape our sexual selves
- The nature and significance of intimacy, touch, love and compassion

Of course, this just skims the surface, so it's mind-boggling to think how little knowledge of sexuality has been incorporated into the educational system for children over the centuries. Again, we can mostly credit religions for such a WO-trocity.

More needs to be done to ensure everyone receives sound information informed by science, not superstition and ignorance, with a focus on such fundamentals as:

- Human reproduction
- The biology of the fertility cycle
- Birth control methods
- Helpful facts, such as 85% of women who have vaginal sex without birth control will become pregnant within a year
- How to use and where to obtain birth control supplies
- How to communicate assertively with a partner about protection

Adults should know a lot more, including the fact that sex;

- Enhances libido in women by increasing vaginal lubrication while improving blood flow and building elasticity
- Improves bladder control in women by building stronger pelvic floor muscles
- Can be enhanced with a variety of mechanical devices that boost sexual arousal, particularly in women, chief among them being a Mercedes-Benz 380sl convertible, according to P.J. O'Rourke
- Lowers blood pressure by burning more calories than watching TV, which essentially burns none at all beyond that required to remain alive
- Reduces pain by releasing endorphins during orgasm
- Improves sleep via the release of prolactin, a relaxation hormone

- Contributes to feel-good sensations, thanks to the release of oxytocin, the hormone that also mitigates anxiety and depression

These are all good reasons for chasing sex but we came across a study recently that, if verifiably true, will revolutionize the skin cream market. It seems researchers at the Royal Edinburgh Hospital in Scotland were able to establish a link between sexuality and youthful appearances. An odd pairing but being the WO-focused social scientists we are, we grabbed our WO-magnifying glasses and peered into this research with more than a little interest.

It seems that a randomized sample of citizens were organized as a panel of judges, assigned to observe participants through one-way mirrors in order to guess the participant ages. These judges had no information on the subjects they observed but their age guesses fascinated the good scientists conducting the study. The researchers found that persons who enjoyed sex on average four times per week, with a steady partner, were perceived to be seven to 12 years younger than their actual age. This finding was explained by the study authors as being attributable to the fact that regular sex promotes the release of testosterone and estrogen, which promotes soft skin and shiny hair.

Could this be true? What if it is? Think of the implications. If I'm having sex four times a week, with a steady partner, and I'm 50 years old but look somewhere between 38 and 43, could I appear between 26 and 36 years of age if I have sex with two steady partners eight times per week. If so, how can I persuade my wife to support this approach for regaining my youthful appearance?

Whether sex makes you look younger or not, it will make you feel WO-filled.

EAT MORE CHOCOLATE

We mean "eat more chocolate" in a metaphorical sense as much as a physical sense. After all, life is short so you don't want to put off the good stuff. You never know, you might never get around to enjoying life's tastiest chocolates.

As to actual chocolate, some forensic anthropologists believe the ancient Aztecs were the first to conclude that chocolate is one of the world's most perfect foods. It's not clear how the Aztecs came to this conclusion but it's true that chocolate does have a lot going for it.

Modern nutritional science has found that chocolate builds immune resistance and helps our bodies fight fatigue. In fact, it offers enough nourishment to sustain a person for an entire day, with nothing else on the menu.

True, chocolate contains a fair amount of sugar and fat. Consuming too much sugar or fat is hazardous but a little each day may be physiologically and psychologically WO-enhancing.

There is ongoing debate regarding the health benefits of chocolate. We know for certain that some fat with a meal helps absorption of fat soluble vitamins and other nutrients, such as vitamin A, D, E, K, the carotenoids in green leafy vegetables and sweet potatoes. Thus, a small amount of chocolate before dinner may be a valuable addition to your diet, not only for its nutrient absorption qualities but also because the fat delays gastric emptying. The latter effect creates a sensation of feeling fuller, resulting in the consumption of smaller meals.

Research also suggests that dark chocolate has heart-protection properties. Cocoa contains high concentrations of flavonoids. Other flavanol-rich foods, such as black tea, green tea, red wine, various fruits and berries have the same antioxidant capacities as chocolate. However, chocolate products that contain more than 70% cocoa appear to be the most beneficial.

There is also some evidence that flavonoids provide cardio-protective effects that defend against oxidation, improve endothelial function, reduce the tendency of blood to clot by improving platelet function and decrease hypertension.

Even better from a WO perspective, Dr Ruth Westheimer suggests "the taste of chocolate is a sensual pleasure in itself, existing in the same world as sex."

Dr Ruth's view is supported by the fact that chocolate stimulates the release of endorphins, the natural brain hormone that generates feelings of pleasure and thus a sense of wellbeing.

Another useful ingredient in chocolate is tryptophan, an essential amino acid the brain employs to produce serotonin, a mood-modulating neurotransmitter that gives rise to feelings of happiness.

There you have it, our case for chocolate based on the reality that the journey is short but making the trip without chocolate could be hazardous to your health and injurious to your WO-pleasures.

TO SMOKE, DRINK OR MASTURBATE

As a public speaker for the past 30 years, Grant has been running a long-term experiment exploring the relationship between audience behaviors and their thought patterns.

"How many people here are smokers?"

A sheepish silence often falls as the large majority of non-smokers turn to place a fixed glare on any perpetrator silly enough to admit such evil doing. Those who do smoke also look around in a mock search designed to throw the self-righteous prosecutors off the track. Rarely does anyone raise their hand.

"Alright then, so how many people here drink alcohol?"

Large numbers quickly raise their hands high, pump their chests and make noises to indicate they drink regularly, signifying that they are socially attuned and part of the crowd. Those few who don't imbibe just roll their eyes in disdain for what they see as drunken bravado.

"Okay, so no smokers and many drinkers."

"Last question, how many people here masturbate?"

At this point the room always erupts into a sea of mirth from embarrassed giggles to uninhibited laughter, as people throw up their hands before rapidly retracting for fear of being caught admitting to such an imagined perversion in public. The noise rises as people turn to each other and question what just happened. Did he really ask that question?

The purpose of the exercise is to show how our brains are so conditioned, over long periods, that one word can change the mood and emotional state of any group.

The next time you're in a group and want a WO-enhancing buzz, just ask everyone what they most like about masturbating.

So how did we get to the point where smokers are vilified, drinkers explode with pride and masturbators slink and recoil?

That's a rhetorical question. We know how societies get to this point. The more interesting question is why do we allow such irrationality to persist?

The big push to ban indoor smoking was fueled by incontrovertible evidence linking smoking with high rates of morbidity and mortality, particularly lung cancer and heart disease.

Besides, the smell was unpleasant for the rest of us. So, if we could reduce smoking, people would live longer and be more productive and less offensive and society's medical costs would fall.

Good idea. Oddly, there is a downside that few experts dare mention: Increased longevity adds to the percentage of people who will suffer the diseases of senescence. Can the already strained medical systems and government payment program manage the added burdens attendant upon fewer smokers?

Logically and economically, if not compassionately, it's better for society that smokers enjoy their two-pack-a-day habits and die early. Instead of glaring at those who point this out, we should be praising their efforts to reduce our economic burden.

Drinking also kills people early but drinking is much more insidious than tobacco smoking. Drinking has social and health consequences much greater than smoking. Yet, alcohol enthusiasts, like those with strong religious beliefs and gun collections, are proud of their attachments.

Those who can't control their drinking kill on the roads, perpetrate domestic violence, fight in the streets, rape and pillage and generally exhibit a series of anti-social behaviors that make life unpleasant for innocents. Yet, we extol drinking as a social virtue, a right of passage to adulthood and a lubricant for people who need extra courage to face reality. The latter often includes the fact that other people don't like them.

We raise our glasses to toast all manner of curious happenings, before a small few slip outside to get some fresh air and a smoke.

All this and we laugh with embarrassment when the subject of masturbation is raised. And if you were caught smoking, drinking and masturbating in the street, you would go to jail for only one of these behaviors.

That's correct; you would be incarcerated for exhibiting the only WO-enhancing behavior while the two WO-inhibiting actions would be seen as quite normal.

Masturbation is relaxing, sometimes exciting and it helps the body release health promoting hormones. More importantly, no one gets hurt.

The WO message here is to promote masturbation. Write to your congressman and demand your freedom to masturbate wherever and whenever you want. You might suggest that your representative set a public example to get the ball rolling, so to speak, even while this long overdue legislation is tied up in Congressional hearings.

Our bottom line advice: Don't smoke or drink but masturbate liberally.

Liberty

FREEDOM

Humans from the beginning of time have had the freedom to think as they like. In this and so many other ways, we are no different from our animal cousins. Our freedom of thought is a gift of nature, not the bounty of gods or states.

What makes us different is something we enjoy that is relatively new to sentient beings, something our brothers and sisters until recently rarely enjoyed and still lack in many areas of the world; the freedom to give voice to thoughts.

This freedom, one we must constantly struggle to protect and expand, is probably the greatest WO of all. It is the equivalent of the lower levels of need such as safety and security that Maslow proclaimed essential foundations for the higher realizations.

Ingersoll claimed "liberty of hand and brain, thought and labor" as his religion, lauding it as "the blossom and fruit of justice, the perfume of mercy."

He saw liberty as "a word hated by kings, loathed by popes." It was a word that represented a concept and a cry for freedom and justice, one that "shattered thrones and altars, left the crown without subjects and the outstretched hand of superstition without alms." For Ingersoll, liberty represented "the seed and soil, the air and light, the dew and rain of progress, love and joy."

LIBERTY THROUGH EDUCATION

Freedom cannot be addressed in the U.S. without acknowledging that slavery and the decades of segregation in the South are ghastly blemishes on American history. The Civil War should have commenced long before the guns went off at Ft. Sumter and the North should have fired first. The bigoted nature of life in the Southern states should have been reformed a century before it actually happened.

The slaves are long gone now, as are their children and many succeeding generations. The injustices to these citizens, ill served by their country, cannot be easily compensated. Their distant descendants have been at a crippling disadvantage since the slave era. Though the issue is raised now and then, financial reparations are no longer a viable proposition, as might have been the case when the Civil War ended.

But, what about education?

Instead of payments for some that would divide many, how about a benefit for everybody needing a boost based on past injustices?

If organized and promoted wisely, educational grants might garner the support of all racial groups while lifting the quality of life for those who still need help.

Instead of money, what about a massive reconstruction plan to educate the less fortunate? And not just for descendants of slaves – all disadvantaged people need help quickly because the trend lines are moving in a very negative direction.

The book, *Room to Grow,* is billed as a manifesto for conservatives, with one chapter author, Peter Wehner, urging Republicans to move beyond the ruinous black and white conviction that our country is divided between all-good and virtuous entrepreneurs (them) and parasitic takers (everybody else). Wehner documents the tribulations of a struggling working middle class and he believes the odds of moving up in America are about half those in more mobile European societies.

Wehner calls for a dynamic process of experimentation to empower families. Other chapter authors propose tax credits and "social guardrails" to guide constructive behaviors, such as early education to promote parenting skills, encourage work and provide urban environments that nurture innovation.

Better education is a logical focus. Famed educator, Robert Balfanz, observes that half of the African-American boys who veer off the path to high school graduation do so in just 660 of more than 12,600 regular and vocational high schools. These students are concentrated in 15 states. While some are in decaying major cities, most are in the South, especially Florida, Georgia and North Carolina. These are the prime candidates for reparation-like educational benefits, as soon as possible.

Let the big data scholars figure out the criteria for eligibility to attend free, high quality, REAL wellness-focused schools from pre-school through high school. It is time to transform public schools for all eligible youth to attend. No charter or parochial or other religious affiliated school should receive public subsidies; parents must be free to send their children to dogma-based institutions if that's what they choose to support. However, no taxpayers should ever be expected to fund close-minded institutions that are hostile to a strict separation of religion and government.

Ingersoll offered seven qualities of Improved Man in an 1892 speech by that title. The second dealt with education. He said this as part of the speech:

> *The Improved Man will be in favor of universal education. He will believe it the duty of every person to shed all the light he can, to the end that no child may be reared in darkness. By education he will mean the gaining of useful knowledge, the development of the mind along the natural paths that lead to human happiness.*

> *He will not waste his time in ascertaining the foolish theories of extinct peoples or in studying the dead languages for the sake of understanding the theologies of ignorance and fear, but he will turn his attention to the affairs of life, and will do his utmost to see to it that every child has an opportunity to learn the demonstrated facts of science, the true history of the world, the great principles of right and wrong applicable to human conduct - the things necessary to the preservation of the individual and of the state, and such arts and industries as are essential to the preservation of all.*

> *He will also endeavor to develop the mind in the direction of the beautiful - of the highest art - so*

*that the palace in which the mind dwells may be en-
riched and rendered beautiful, to the end that these
stones, called facts, may be changed into statues.*

That's what a REAL wellness curriculum would advance throughout the formative years.

Such education would do the things noted in the *Improved Man*
lecture. It would guide students into alignment with nature, with
the conditions of wellbeing and with concern for the wellbeing of
others.

Children and young adults would learn to discern the facts in nature and their connections with others around the world. They
would be educated human beings of an Ingersollian nature.

> *The educated man knows something that he can
> use, not only for the benefit of himself, but for the
> benefit of others. Every skilled mechanic, every good
> farmer, every man who knows some of the real facts
> in nature that touch him, is to that extent an edu-
> cated man. The skilled mechanic and the intelligent
> farmer may not be what we call 'scholars,' and what
> we call scholars may not be educated men.*

> *Man is in constant need. He must protect himself
> from cold and heat, from sun and storm. He needs
> food and raiment for the body, and he needs what
> we call art for the development and gratification of
> his brain. Beginning with what are called the nec-
> essaries of life, he rises to what are known as the
> luxuries, and the luxuries become necessaries, and
> above luxuries he rises to the highest wants of the
> soul.*

The man who is fitted to take care of himself, in the conditions he may be placed, is, in a very important sense, an educated man. The savage who understands the habits of animals, who is a good hunter and fisher, is a man of education, taking into consideration his circumstances. The graduate of a university who cannot take care of himself, no matter how much he may have studied, is not an educated man.

In our time, an educated man, whether a mechanic, a farmer, or one who follows a profession, should know something about what the world has discovered. He should have an idea of the outlines of the sciences. He should have read a little, at least, of the best that has been written. He should know something of mechanics, a little about politics, commerce, and metaphysics; and in addition to all this, he should know how to make something. His hands should be educated, so that he can, if necessary, supply his own wants by supplying the wants of others.

There are mental misers - men who gather learning all their lives and keep it to themselves. They are worse than hoarders of gold, because when they die their learning dies with them, while the metal miser is compelled to leave his gold for others.

The first duty of man is to support himself, to see to it that he does not become a burden.

His next duty is to help others if he has a surplus, and if he really believes they deserve to be helped.

It is not necessary to have what is called a university education in order to be useful or to be happy, any more than it is necessary to be rich, to be happy. Great wealth is a great burden, and to have more than you can use, is to care for more than you want. The happiest are those who are prosperous, and who by reasonable endeavor can supply their reasonable wants and have a little surplus year by year for the winter of their lives.

So, it is no use to learn thousands and thousands of useless facts, or to fill the brain with unspoken tongues. This is burdening yourself with more than you can use. The best way is to learn the useful.

We all know that men in moderate circumstances can have just as comfortable houses as the richest, just as comfortable clothing, just as good food. They can see just as fine paintings, just as marvelous statues, and they can hear just as good music. They can attend the same theaters and the same operas. They can enjoy the same sunshine, and above all, can love and be loved just as well as kings and millionaires.

So the conclusion of the whole matter is, that he is educated who knows how to take care of himself; and that the happy man is the successful man, and that it is only a burden to have more than you want, or to learn those things that you cannot use.

These words were printed in The High School Register, Omaha, Nebraska in January, 1891 and they would serve us well today as objectives for educating our children, particularly those who need their government's support for past injustices in the provision of a decent education.

FREEDOM OF SPEECH

Save for Don's early years as a student in Catholic school classrooms, governed by nuns and Christian Brothers, we really don't know what it must be like to live under a totalitarian system that restricts speech and punishes unapproved expression severely.

However, we can imagine that it's not much fun so, as with Ingersoll, liberty is definitely our religion.

> *I am a believer in liberty. That is my religion — to give to every other human being every right that I claim for myself and I grant to every other human being, not the right — because it is his right — but instead of granting I declare that it is his right, to attack every doctrine that I maintain, to answer every argument that I may urge — in other words, he must have absolute freedom of speech. (Spoken in Ingersoll's roles as defense counsel at the trial of C.B. Reynolds for blasphemy, May 1887)*

Freedom of speech sounds great but there are prerequisites. If neglected, freedom of speech can become more a slogan than a reality and not enjoyed or embraced to the Ingersoll standard of liberty.

One prerequisite for speech freely communicated is an educated citizenry because it takes considerable reinforcement over time to appreciate and become accustomed to speech with which we don't agree.

It is a bit of a paradox to agree in principle with liberty but to take offense when it is exercised in ways not quite to your liking. Theodore Roosevelt had wise words to offer on this point, even though doing so ran contrary to his own interests as president:

> *To announce that there must be no criticism of the President or that we are to stand by the President, right or wrong, is not only unpatriotic and servile but is morally treasonable to the American public.*

Thomas Jefferson expressed this sentiment even more strenuously when he said:

> *Dissent is the highest form of patriotism.*

You would certainly want a speaker at a public forum to give everyone their best counsel, to be comfortable and welcomed to hit you with their best shot, to fire away and thus provide the best lessons and insights they have to offer. As George Orwell suggests:

> *If liberty means anything at all, it means the right to tell people what they do not want to hear.*

How many dissenters can we readily identify whom we admire? If you are a genuine enthusiast for free speech, you should have no trouble rattling off any number of such characters. One who quickly comes to our minds is the late, much lamented, Christopher Hitchens:

> *My own opinion is enough for me and I claim the right to have it defended against any consensus, any majority, anywhere, any place, any time. And anyone who disagrees with this can pick a number, get in line, and kiss my ass.*

Most people burdened by the misfortune to be oppressed under totalitarian governments, including theocracies, learn to keep their inconsistencies with unchallengeable truths to themselves, a custom about which Euripides had this to say:

> This is slavery, not to speak one's thought. (The Phoenician Women)

In addition to a democratic state, a well-educated citizenry and a culture of tolerance for diverse opinions, a sense of humor is extremely helpful. In nearly half the world today, people are not inclined to find irreverent jokes or cartoons acceptable; in some dictatorships, people can be killed over a perceived insult to an imaginary being.

Oscar Wilde's sentiments about freedom of speech would not go over well in Saudi Arabia:

> I may not agree with you but I will defend to the death your right to make an ass of yourself.

Naturally, there are some limits on everything, including speech. There cannot be freedom to say that which brings actual harm or damage to others, or words that meet the libel test.

Freedom of speech requires a citizenry capable of knowing where lines are drawn by citizen consent. Jim C. Hines once observed that freedom of speech does not protect you from the consequences of saying stupid shit.

Unfettered expression is important for another reason: It represents a mother lode of possibilities for exuberance. The art of creative expression uninhibited by constraints of censorship, the fear of giving offense, blaspheming or violating speech codes enables

WOs large and small, ephemeral and long lasting. Such speech, whether in books, e-mails, letters, conversations, phone or Skype chats are part of a bountiful harvest from the fields of spontaneity.

Without free expression, art would be poorer. Consider the books banned, the films censored and the music suppressed even in recent times. Fortunately, these anti-liberty impulses have been overcome in most Western nations, though retrograde efforts to control speech continue in the backwoods of Alabama, Mississippi and well, pretty much everywhere in the South and most Red states. It is more true than not that the GOP is becoming more "God's Own Party" than the Grand Old Party.

So far, except perhaps at the Texas and Kansas School Board levels, reason prevails and liberty is restored. Personally, we'd be more than a little disappointed if censorship prevented artistic expression that religious interests found offensive; perhaps a play for example, like *The Book of Mormon* or the song "Imagine" by John Lennon:

> Imagine there's no heaven
> It's easy if you try
> No hell below us
> Above us only sky
> Imagine all the people
> Living for today...

You can easily understand why seekers of REAL wellness and multiple WOs take liberty in general, and freedom of speech in particular, so seriously.

The takeaway message for a fun life in a meaningless world; encourage freedom of speech at every opportunity, even if some of it might not be to your liking.

What Robert Green Ingersoll said of reason also applies to freedom of speech:

> *I admit that (freedom of speech) is a small and feeble flame, a flickering torch by stumblers carried in the starless night, blown and flared by passion's storms and yet, it is the only light. Extinguish it and nought remains.*

STAYING VIGILANT

We are constantly inspired by the words of great women and men who lived before our time, as well as the heroes of liberty who are still part of our world today. Many observations of consequence to WO seekers can be found in literature of many kinds including, as discussed throughout, the words of Robert Green Ingersoll (1833-1899).

In the spirit of Ingersoll, we have a few suggestions for modest initiatives to help you loosen inhibitions that might still be clinging from years of non-WO supportive customs, cultures, relatives or friends.

- Develop a conscious appreciation of remaining aware at all times to the importance of self-emancipation from society's unrelenting temptations to control your thinking, your speech and your actions
- Know that freedom is a battle to be waged constantly, even by those of us fortunate to live in lands that give at least lip service to liberty
- Think of liberty as your ally and a companion of multiple WOs on the road of REAL wellnesßs
- Realize that absolute freedom to do whatever you like, regardless of the consequences for others, is as unreasonable

as are the totalitarian limits on freedom that most of us rightly abhor

Ingersoll believed that "life is poor enough at best; no one should fail to pick up every jewel of joy that can be found in his path."

Similarly, we think freedom is rare and fragile, that no one can afford to miss an opportunity to defend and advance human rights at every turn.

To think, speak and act freely are essential prerequisites for REAL wellness functioning.

WORDS EXTOLLING LIBERTY TO PONDER AND EMBRACE

> *Men fear thought as they fear nothing else on earth - more than ruin, more even than death. Thought is subversive and revolutionary, destructive and terrible, thought is merciless to privilege, established institutions and comfortable habits; thought is anarchic and lawless, indifferent to authority, careless of the well-tried wisdom of the ages. Thought looks into the pit of hell and is not afraid. Thought is great and swift and free, the light of the world and the chief glory of man.*
> **Bertrand Russell**

> *Emancipate yourselves from mental slavery. None but ourselves can free our minds.* **Bob Marley**

> *I do this real moron thing and it's called thinking. And apparently I'm not a very good American because I like to form my own opinions.* **George Carlin**

Blind belief in authority is the greatest enemy of truth. **Albert Einstein**

It is dangerous to be right in matters on which the established authorities are wrong. **Voltaire**

Libraries should be open to all, except the censor. **John F. Kennedy**

The country was in peril; he was jeopardizing his traditional rights of freedom and independence by daring to exercise them. **Joseph Heller**

It is very nearly impossible to become an educated person in a country so distrustful of the independent mind. **James Baldwin**

Ideas are far more powerful than guns. We don't let our people have guns. Why should we let them have ideas? **Joseph Stalin**

If a believer demands that I, as a nonbeliever, observe his taboos in the public domain, he is not asking for my respect but for my submission. **Flemming Rose**

The moment you say that any idea system is sacred, whether it's a religious belief system or a secular ideology, the moment you declare a set of ideas to be immune from criticism, satire, derision or contempt, freedom of thought becomes impossible. **Salman Rushdie**

You can't pick and choose which types of freedom you want to defend. You must defend all of it or be against all of it. **Scott Howard Phillips**

Restriction of free thought and free speech is the most dangerous of all subversions. It is the one un-American act that could most easily defeat us.
William O Douglas

FREE TO BREED AND FEED THE SEETHING MASSES

People the world over, except possibly the Chinese in recent decades, have been free to breed like rabbits cheered on by religions.

Thus, the population bomb has become ever more powerful. Despite vast improvements in developed nations, with reduced infant and childhood mortality through improved disease controls, public education, advanced medical care, sanitation and other gains in the quality of civilization, there remain vast areas of the earth where conditions remain medieval.

While we are enthusiastic about maximum freedoms, we don't go to *reducio ad absurdum* levels with this posture. We think it's not really "freedom" when the liberties taken by some diminish the rights of others or lower their quality of life. Such is the case with unfettered freedom to breed beyond the point wherein societies can protect quality of life prospects for all.

We've noticed that some forums on environment and sustainability ignore or give scant attention to the planetary elephant in the room; namely, overpopulation.

Perhaps this neglect explains how mega-corporations can excuse their lack of accountability for well-established environmental worries. Ignoring population expansion enables big business to burn resources at unsustainable rates. The leaders of extraction and other industries evidently assume that their shareholders expect them to downplay future crises of global warming, loss of arable lands, clean water shortages and other dwindling energy resources as lesser concerns than immediate reductions in their continued huge profit margins.

Unfortunately, these great problems today and looming disasters tomorrow are rooted in the unfettered population explosion.

So, how can the earth sustain the 9.6 billion people the Pew Research Center (2014) project will inhabit the earth by 2050? How many governments, institutions or other forces with the power to change public awareness and action are likely to take leadership in addressing the explosive power of the thermonuclear population bomb?

One thing seems certain; the environmentalists, economists and others concerned about the population threat will get no help from fundamentalist religions. The Catholic Church maintains a "populate or perish" mindset, fortified by "the meek shall inherit the earth" sound bites. The Vatican continues to oppose not only the right to choose abortion but also contraception. In poor, over-populated and starving areas of the world, Catholic doctrine even opposes free condoms for the poor. All other religions are just as destructive or useless.

Where is the population tipping point? What possible role can the Liberty element of REAL wellness play in mitigating the tsunami of rising horrors? What could possibly bring a sea change in attitudes to help abate out-of-control population increases?

Back in the 1970's, Paul and Anne Ehrlich made an interesting case in *The Population Bomb* for the idea that overpopulation would eventually cause widespread famine throughout the world. The fact this forecast has not yet come to pass only reduces public appreciation of the population argument the Ehrlich's tried to express.

So far, global death rates continue to decline and populations continue to grow, with people gaining access to plentiful calories as science devises ever more clever ways, through gene manipulation, to grow more food on increasingly marginal lands.

Along with the smarts of science denying an Ehrich type famine, Nobel Prize winning Indian economist, Amartya Sen, suggests democratic nations, with a free press, also never seem to suffer from extended famines.

India, with almost 1.3 billion people and a Total Fertility Rate (TFR) around 2.6, has a high absolute number of malnourished children. Yet, the rates of malnutrition and poverty have declined in that country from approximately 90% at the time of India's independence from British colonial rule to less than 40% today. Tellingly, since India became a democracy, there have been no recorded famines. Perhaps this suggests an unrecognized benefit of freedom at both a national and personal level.

Perhaps a combination of science and freedom marked by democratic decision-making can boost hopes for feeding a burgeoning population. But, can the two elements also address the paradoxical problem of resource depletion brought on by the demands of a rising middle class in once impoverished nations?

Let us hope so. If not, we will have fewer opportunities than we do now to enjoy WOs and REAL wellness. Our only hopes rest with science and reason. History shows that liberty can provide abundance while famine is the domain of tyranny.

Luminary Lane

A WALK DOWN LUMINARY LANE

Many of the greatest minds in history have taken a rational, WO filled view of life. The sheer number of luminaries who favor science over religion is encouraging to freethinkers.

Perhaps, in time, reason will overtake faith. When and if that ever happens, our species will better appreciate and look after the Earth's extraordinary natural wonders. What's more, we all will better appreciate the wonder of our chance existence.

This walk down our REAL wellness Lane of Luminescence features 18 women and men who have contributed multiple WO-inspiring perspectives. We offer a few of their words for the insights they evoke and to encourage you to explore more of their life works.

Isaac Asimov (1920-1992)

A prolific author of more than 470 books on science and science fiction, Asimov followed what he called "the Asimovian Law of Composition." Writing from 6:30 am until 10 pm, seven days a week, he produced, on average, 12 books annually. His output was said to be encyclopedic, ranging from "Asimov's Guide to the Bible" (1968) to "Asimov's Annotated Paradise Lost" (1974).

I am Jewish in the sense that if an Arab wanted to throw a rock at a Jew, I would qualify as a target as far as he was concerned. However, I do not practice Judaism or any other religion.

I must say that I stand amazed at the highly intelligent people who have taken so much of the Bible so seriously.

I would not be satisfied to have my kids choose to be religious without trying to argue them out of it, just as I would not be satisfied to have them decide to smoke regularly or engage in any other practice I considered detrimental to mind or body.

I am prejudiced against religion because I know the history of religion, and it is the history of human misery and of black crimes.

I believe in evidence. I believe in observation, measurement and reasoning, confirmed by independent observers. I'll believe anything, no matter how wild and ridiculous, if there is evidence for it. The wilder and more ridiculous something is, however, the firmer and more solid the evidence will have to be.

Madalyn Murray O'Hair (1919 - 1995)

Madalyn Murray O'Hair was a champion of secularism. Time magazine called Madalyn Murray O'Hair the most hated woman in America during her reign as a leading secularist in the second half of the 20th century. Her unyielding and, to most, abrasive defense of the wall separating government from religion was as effective as it was controversial. She relished every opportunity to provoke the faithful and challenge public officials who illegally granted religion special privilege in American life. School prayer was the first of many issues that brought Madalyn to public attention when she objected to Bible readings in the Baltimore public schools.

O'Hair founded American Atheists and debated religious leaders on a variety of issues across the land. She annoyed nearly everyone, including fellow religious skeptics and her life truly was an unhappy mess. She is credited with helping put a halt to plans that would have had astronaut Buzz Aldrin staging a televised communion on the moon. She also blocked a Texas law that would have required public officials to affirm belief in a Supreme Being. O'Hair tried, like many other atheists since, to get "In God We Trust" off coins and to prevent the pope from saying mass on the Mall in Washington, D.C. She also took legal action in efforts to put a stop to tax exemptions for churches.

> *I'll tell you what you did with atheists for about 1500 years. You outlawed them from the universities or any teaching careers, besmirched their reputations, banned or burned their books or their writings of any kind, drove them into exile, humiliated them, seized their properties, arrested them for blasphemy. You dehumanized them with beatings and exquisite torture, gouged out their eyes,*

slit their tongues, stretched, crushed, or broke their limbs, tore off their breasts if they were women, crushed their scrotums if they were men, imprisoned them, stabbed them, disemboweled them, hanged them, burnt them alive. And you have nerve enough to complain to me that I laugh at you?

This religion gives you goals, which are outside of reality. It enriches your fantasy life with ugliness. It fills you with ideas of guilt over the most common human experiences -- usually related to sex. In this room, right now, each of you, in your own lives, has agonized over the fact that you have masturbated. Masturbation isn't sinful. If it feels good -- do it. You have my blessing and you yourself know how it relaxes you.

People say, `So what? It's just a little cross.' What if it were a little swastika?

Atheism may be defined as the mental attitude, which unreservedly accepts the supremacy of reason and aims at establishing a lifestyle and ethical outlook verifiable by experience and the scientific method, independent of all arbitrary assumptions of authority and creeds.

Ayaan Hirsi Ali (1969 - present)

A Somali-born American activist, writer and politician, Ali is known for her views on Islam, female genital mutilation, women's rights and atheism. Author of two bestselling books, *Infidel: My Life* and *Nomad: from Islam to America*, she was named by Time magazine as one of the 100 most influential people in the world in 2005. Ali has several other distinctions and awards, including a free speech prize from the Danish newspaper Jyllands-Posten, the Swedish Liberal Party's Democracy Prize and the Moral Courage Award for commitment to conflict resolution, ethics and world citizenship.

All life is problem solving. There are no absolutes; progress comes through critical thought. Reason, not obedience, should guide our lives. Though it took centuries to crumble, the entire ossified cage of European social hierarchy - from kings to serfs, and between men and women, all of it shored up by the Catholic Church - was destroyed by this thought.

When a 'Life of Brian' comes out with Muhammad in the lead role, directed by an Arab equivalent of Theo van Gogh, it will be a huge step forward.

Tolerance of intolerance is cowardice.

George Carlin (1937 - 2008)

An outspoken comedian who won two Grammys, Carlin was arrested in Milwaukee in 1972 for performing his now immortal "Seven Dirty Words You Can't Say on Radio or Television" routine. He inspired the Freedom From Religion Foundation's "Emperor Has No Clothes Award" and was the first to receive that honor. It recognizes public figures who "tell it like it is" about religion. He was the first host of "Saturday Night Live" (1975) and appeared in 11 HBO specials.

When evolution is outlawed, only outlaws will evolve.

I don't have pet peeves — I have major psychotic fucking hatreds!

Think of how stupid the average person is, and realize half of them are stupider than that.

I'm completely in favor of the separation of church and state. My idea is that these two institutions screw us up enough on their own, so both of them together is certain death.

Religion has convinced people that there's an invisible man...living in the sky, who watches everything you do every minute of every day. And the invisible man has a list of ten specific things he doesn't want you to do. And if you do any of these things, he will send you to a special place, of burning and fire and smoke and torture and anguish for you to live forever, and suffer and burn and scream until the end of time. But he loves you. He loves you and he needs money.

Anne Nicol Gaylor (1926 - present)

As editor of the Middleton Times Tribune, Anne Nicole Gaylor editorialized from 1997 for legalized abortion. Requests from pregnant women in desperate straits led Ms Gaylor into volunteer activism for feminist rights. She founded the ZPG Abortion Referral Service in 1970, which resulted in 20,000-plus referrals for birth control, abortion and sterilization over an initial five year period. Two years later, she co-founded a charity to assist low-income women seeking abortions; a service that helped 14,000 women over a 32 year period. In 1976, Ms Gaylor and two others, including her daughter Annie Laurie, created the Freedom From Religion Foundation (FFRF) for the promotion of free thought and separation of state and church. Today, FFRF has over 21,000 members and a distinguished record of legal actions.

Nothing fails like prayer.

There were many groups working for women's rights but none of them dealt with the root cause of women's oppression - religion.

There are no gods, no devils, no angels, no heaven or hell. There is only our natural world. Religion is but myth and superstition that hardens hearts and enslaves minds.

Wendy Kaminer (1950 - present)

A graduate of Smith College in 1971 and Boston University Law School in 1975, Kaminer spent her first years practicing law before switching to journalism in 1991. Her eight books include, *Sleeping with Extra-Terrestrials: The Rise of Irrationalism, Free for All: Defending Liberty in America Today* and *Perils of Piety.* She has received many recognitions of a major nature, including the Extraordinary Merit Media Award from the National Women's Political Caucus and a Guggenheim fellowship. The focus of Kaminer's work includes atheism and state/church issues, the harm of religions influence on politics, civil liberties, psychology and the law.

Atheists generate about as much sympathy as pedophiles. But, while pedophilia may at least be characterized as a disease, atheism is a choice, a willful rejection of beliefs to which vast majorities of people cling.

The magical thinking encouraged by any belief in the supernatural, combined with the vilification of rationality and skepticism, is more conducive to conspiracy theories than it is to productive political debate.

I don't care if religious people consider me amoral because I lack their beliefs in God. I do, however, care deeply about efforts to turn religious beliefs into law, and those efforts benefit greatly from the conviction that individually and collectively, we cannot be good without God.

Christopher Hitchens (1949 - 2011)

Born in England and educated at Cambridge and Oxford, Hitchens worked as a book reviewer (London Times), editor (The Atlantic Monthly and Vanity Fair) and a foreign correspondent, covering events in 60 countries on five continents. He moved to the U.S. and became a US citizen while writing many books, none better known than *God Is Not Great* (2007). Among his favorite targets were President Clinton, the Pope, Mother Theresa and progressive critics of his pro-Iraqi war positions.

Gullibility and credulity are considered undesirable qualities in every department of human life - except religion . . . Why are we praised by godly men for surrendering our 'godly gift' of reason when we cross their mental thresholds? . . . Atheism strikes me as morally superior, as well as intellectually superior, to religion. Since it is obviously inconceivable that all religions can be right, the most reasonable conclusion is that they are all wrong.

Take the risk of thinking for yourself, much more happiness, truth, beauty, and wisdom will come to you that way.

If religious instruction were not allowed until the child had attained the age of reason, we would be living in a quite different world.

Matilda Joslyn Gage (1826-1898)

Ms Gage distinguished herself as a suffragette, abolitionist, Native American activist, secularist and feminist. She worked closely with Susan B. Anthony and Elizabeth Cady Stanton as an eloquent spokesperson for the then outrageous idea that women had a natural right to vote. Matilda served as President of the National Woman Suffrage Association and in 1890 organized the Woman's National Liberal Union devoted to separation of church and state. Over a century ago, Gage identified the church as the root cause of the oppression of women and also warned about a danger that confronts the country today, namely, a union of Catholics and Protestants attempting to put God in the Constitution and attack secular schools.

It is the church and not the state, to which the teaching of woman's inferiority is due: it is the church, which primarily commanded the obedience of woman to man. It is the church, which stamps with religious authority the political and domestic degradation of woman.

There is a word sweeter than mother, home or heaven. That word is liberty.

In order to help preserve the very life of the Republic, it is imperative that women should unite upon a platform of opposition to the teaching and aim of that ever most unscrupulous enemy of freedom - the Church.

During the ages, no rebellion has been of like importance with that of woman against the tyranny of the church and state; none has had its far reaching effects. We note its beginning; its progress will overthrow every existing form of these institutions; its end will be a regenerated world.

Robert G. Ingersoll (1833 - 1899)

Ingersoll, the "Great Agnostic" and a REAL wellness pioneer, was the best known advocate of free thought in 19th century America. The son of a minister, he became an attorney via apprenticeship and, in 1887, was appointed the first Attorney General of Illinois. He served in the Union Army as a colonel in the Civil War, fighting in the Battle of Shiloh. He came to national prominence with his presidential nomination speech for James G. Blaine at the national convention of the Republican Party in 1876. He helped elect three U.S. presidents with his spellbinding oratory. Today, Ingersoll is revered by secularists for his encyclopedic body of work, including speeches that were delivered before capacity audiences in nearly every state in the Union, over a 35-year period, following the Civil War.

His lectures addressed contributions of Shakespeare, Voltaire, Paine and Burns but the largest crowds came out to hear him denounce the bible and religion in general and the infamous doctrine of hell, superstition and all dogma-based barriers to happiness, liberty and reason in particular.

Happiness is the only good; reason the only torch; justice the only worship, humanity the only religion and love the only priest.

Blasphemy is the word that the majority hisses into the ears of the few. Each church has accused nearly every other of being a blasphemer. The Catholics called Martin Luther a blasphemer and Martin Luther called Copernicus a blasphemer. Pious ignorance always regards intelligence as a kind of blasphemy. Some of the greatest men of the world, some of the best, have been put to death for blasphemy. After every argument of the church has been answered, has been refuted, then the church cries, "Blasphemy!" Blasphemy is what an old mistake says of a newly discovered truth. Blasphemy is the bulwark of religious prejudice. Blasphemy is the breastplate of the heartless. The Infinite cannot be blasphemed.

Who can over estimate the progress of the world if all the money wasted in superstition could be used to enlighten, elevate and civilize mankind?

If you wish depth, genius, imagination, taste, reason, sensibility, philosophy, elevation, originality, nature, intellect, fancy, rectitude, facility, flexibility, precision, art, abundance, variety, fertility, warmth, magic, charm, grace, force, an "eagle sweep" of vision, vast understanding, instruction, rich tone, excellent, urbanity, suavity, delicacy, correctness, purity, clearness, éloquence, harmony, brillance, rapidity, gaiety, pathos, sublimity and universality, perfection indeed, behold Voltaire.

Butterfly McQueen (1911 - 1995)

A dancer turned actress, Thelma "Butterfly" McQueen is best known for playing "Prissy" in *Gone with the Wind* (1939). She acted in twenty other movies and television into the 1950s. During World War II, she made many appearances on the Armed Forces Broadcast "Jubilee" as a comedienne. Butterfly was a nearly life-long atheist. She retired from acting because studio executives felt she was insufficiently deferential for a black woman and so she often worked in service jobs including, ironically, as a maid, as a salesperson at Macy's, a taxi dispatcher, running a snack shop and as a seamstress. She graduated in 1974, at age 64, from New York City College with a bachelor's degree in political science.

> *As my ancestors are free from slavery, I am free from the slavery of religion.*

> *I'm an atheist and Christianity appears to me to be the most absurd imposture of all the religions and I'm puzzled that so many people can't see through a religion that encourages irresponsibility and bigotry.*

> *They say the streets are going to be beautiful in heaven. Well, I'm trying to make the streets beautiful here. . . . When it's clean and beautiful, I think America is heaven. And some people are hell.*

Bill Maher (1956 - present)

Host of *Real Time with Bill Maher* on HBO, Maher wrote four best-sellers; *True Story* in 2005, *Does Anybody Have a Problem with That? Politically Incorrect's Greatest Hits* in 1997, *When You Ride Alone, You Ride With Bin Laden* in 2002 and *New Rules: Polite Musings from a Timid Observer* in 2006.

Maher has performed nine comedy specials for HBO, starred on Comedy Central and performs stand-up comedy shows annually in Las Vegas. He specializes in satirizing Republicans and warning of the dangers of political religion. His movie "Religulous" (2008) is the seventh-highest grossing documentary of all time.

New rule: If churches don't have to pay taxes, they also can't call the fire department when they catch fire. Sorry reverend, that's one of those services that goes along with paying in. I'll use the fire department I pay for. You can pray for rain.

If you have a few hundred followers and you let some of them molest children, they call you a cult leader. If you have a billion, they call you Pope.

I hate religion. I think it's a neurological disorder.

When I hear from people that religion doesn't hurt anything, I say, really? Well besides wars, the Crusades, the Inquisitions, 9-11, ethnic cleansing, the suppression of women, the suppression of homosexuals, fatwas, honor killings, suicide bombings, arranged marriages to minors, human sacrifice, burning witches, and systematic sex with children, I have a few little quibbles. And I forgot blowing up girl schools in Afghanistan.

Thomas Paine (1737 - 1809)

Born in England, Paine became a founder of the American nation. He wrote *Common Sense* in 1776, which is credited with sparking the American Revolution and the classic criticism of the bible, *The Age of Reason* in 1792.

Paine repudiated the divine origin of Christianity on grounds that it was too "absurd for belief, too impossible to convince and too inconsistent to practice."

> *I believe that religious duties consist in doing justice, loving mercy, and endeavoring to make our fellow creatures happy. I do not believe in the creed professed by the Jewish Church, by the Roman Church, by the Greek Church, by the Turkish Church, by the Protestant Church, nor by any church that I know of. My own mind is my own church. Organized religion was set up to terrify and enslave and to monopolize power and profit.*

> *Whenever we read the obscene stories, the voluptuous debaucheries, the cruel and tortuous executions, the unrelenting vindictiveness, with which more than half the Bible is filled it would be more consistent that we call it the word of a demon than the word of God. It is a history of wickedness that has served to corrupt and brutalize.*

Carl Sagan (1934 - 1996)

Carl Sagan was a professor of astronomy and space science and director of the Laboratory for Planetary Studies at Cornell University.

He was the great popularizer of science who produced and narrated *Cosmos*, a PBS series watched by 500 million people in 60 countries that won Emmy and Peabody awards. His 20 books, including *Cosmos, The Dragons of Eden, Pale Blue Dot* and *The Demon-Haunted World: Science as a Candle in the Dark* were all best sellers. The latter was his most notable take down critique of religion.

Sagan also co-produced the movie *Contact* and played a leading role in NASA's Mariner, Viking, Voyager and Galileo expeditions to other planets. His wife, Ann Druyan, wrote an account of his struggle with bone marrow cancer as an epilogue to Sagan's last book, *Billions and Billions: Thoughts on Life and Death at the Brink of the Millennium,* published posthumously in 1997.

> *If some good evidence for life after death were announced, I'd be eager to examine it; but it would have to be real scientific data, not mere anecdote. As with the face on Mars and alien abductions, better the hard truth, I say, than the comforting fantasy. And in the final tolling it often turns out that the facts are more comforting than the fantasy.*
>
> *For me, it is far better to grasp the Universe as it really is than to persist in delusion, however satisfying and reassuring.*
>
> *But the fact that some geniuses were laughed at does not imply that all who are laughed at are geniuses. They laughed at Columbus, they laughed at Fulton, they laughed at the Wright brothers. But they also laughed at Bozo the Clown.*
>
> *In every country, we should be teaching our children the scientific method and the reasons for a Bill of*

Rights. With it comes a certain decency, humility and community spirit. In the demon-haunted world that we inhabit by virtue of being human, this may be all that stands between us and the enveloping darkness.

Elizabeth Cady Stanton (1815 - 1902)

Elizabeth Cady Stanton is viewed as the founding mother of the feminist movement. Her issues were women's subjugation and religion's role in keeping women subordinate. A suffrage plank she introduced at the historic Seneca Falls convention in 1848 won endorsement and galvanized women for the next 72 years. In her diary, she noted that her beliefs were "grounded on science, common sense and love of humanity, not fears of the torments of hell and promises of the joys of heaven." She described how "the bible was hurled at us from every side" in a history of the early movement. Nearly every speech Stanton wrote condemned religious dogma. She is also fondly remembered by contemporary secularists for writing *The Woman's Bible* in 1895.

The Church is a terrible engine of oppression, especially as concerns woman.

I have endeavored to dissipate these religious superstitions from the minds of women and base their faith on science and reason, where I found for myself at least that peace and comfort I could never find in the Bible and the church. . . the less they believe, the better for their own happiness and development.

For fifty years the women of this nation have tried to dam up this deadly stream that poisons all their lives but thus far they have lacked the insight or courage to follow it back to its source and there strike the blow at the fountain of all tyranny, religious superstition, priestly power and the canon law.

Mark Twain (Samuel Clemens 1835 - 1910)

America's iconoclastic humorist, Mark Twain wrote *Tom Sawyer*, *The Adventures of Huckleberry Finn* and other world renowned classics. He said he was poor as a boy but didn't know it and everybody was comfortable and did know it. His mother, Jane Lampton Clemens, was an advocate for the downtrodden and "could be beguiled into saying a soft word for the devil himself," Twain recalled.

In the 1884 novel *Huck Finn*, Huck decides it is better to be damned to hell rather than betray his friend, a runaway slave, observing: "Hain't we got all the fools in town on our side? And hain't that a big enough majority in any town?" Twain's *The War Prayer*, written in 1905 but not published until 1923, is a scathing indictment of war and religious hypocrisy.

Faith is believing what you know ain't so.

I cannot see how a man of any large degree of humorous perception can ever be religious - except he purposely shut the eyes of his mind and keep them shut by force.

Man is the only religious animal. He is the only animal that has the True Religion -several of them. He is the only animal that loves his neighbor as himself and cuts his throat, if his theology isn't straight. He has made a graveyard of the globe in trying his honest best to smooth his brother's path to happiness and heaven.

Voltaire (Francois-Marie Arouet - 1694 – 1778)

Born in Paris, Voltaire first came to public attention as a poet, a playwright and a political activist of the Enlightenment. Imprisoned in 1718 in the Bastille, he was released upon agreeing to move to London. There he wrote *Lettres philosophiques* in 1733, leading his enemies in France to regret letting him go. The book galvanized French reform and satirized religion.

Voltaire wrote *Candide* in 1759 and devoted his work to challenging Christianity, which he called "the infamous thing," focusing in particular on transubstantiation, miracles and biblical contradictions.

> *Christianity is the most ridiculous, the most absurd and bloody religion that has ever infected the world.*

> *A true god surely cannot have been born of a girl, nor died on the gibbet, nor be eaten in a piece of dough or inspired books filled with contradictions, madness and horror.*

> *Atheism is the vice of a few intelligent people. The truths of religion are never so well understood as by those who have lost the power of reasoning.*

Neil deGrasse Tyson (1958 - present)

While a young staff scientist at the Hayden Planetarium at the American Museum of Natural History (1994–1995), Tyson wrote the *Universe* essays for Natural History (1995–2005). He has hosted PBS's *NOVA scienceNOW* since 2006. Tyson has served on NASA's advisory council and as the director of the Hayden Planetarium. His nine books include *Origins: Fourteen Billion Years of Cosmic Evolution* (2005), *Death by Black Hole: And Other Cosmic Quandaries* (2007), and *The Sky is Not the Limit: Adventure of an Urban Astrophysicist* (2000). He recently starred in the new version of *Cosmos,* produced by Carl Sagan's widow, Ann Druyan.

Carl Sagan befriended Tyson before and during his studies at Cornell University where Dr Sagan was a professor.

> *I have yet to see a successful prediction about the physical world that was inferred or extrapolated from the content of any religions documents.*

> *Intelligent design is a philosophy of ignorance. You cannot build a program of discovery on the assumption that nobody is smart enough to figure out the answer to a problem. I don't want students who could make the next major breakthrough in renewable energy sources or space travel to have been taught that anything they don't understand, and that nobody yet understands, is divinely constructed and therefore beyond their intellectual capacity. The day that happens, Americans will just sit in awe of what we don't understand, while we watch the rest of the world boldly go where no mortal has gone before.*

> *Let there be no doubt that as they are currently practiced, there is no common ground between science and religion.*

Vashti McCollum (1912 - 2006)

Vashti McCollum endured the wrath of the loving faithful, including death threats, harassed children, murder of the family cat, job loss and more, for challenging school prayer in the public schools and eventually winning the Supreme Court case that put a stop to religious education in public schools in America. This 1948 ruling remains in force to this day. Her book, *One Woman's Fight* (1953), was a best seller and propelled her career as a free thought leader. Ms McCollum served two terms as president of the American Humanist Association and she was featured in a PBS documentary entitled, *The Lord Is Not on Trial Here.* The title was inspired by an incident during court hearings when a Bible-toting man confronted the school board's attorney, announcing that he was there to testify for the Lord. The attorney replied, "The Lord, sir, is not on trial here today."

To their credit, the Baptist Joint Committee submitted an amicus brief to the Court in support of McCollum, saying, "We must not allow our religious fervor to blind us to the essential fact that no religious faith is secure when it meshes its authority with that of the state."

> *Between being praised and persecuted, condoned and condemned, I might understandably have become bewildered, particularly at the brand of ethics sometimes displayed by the staunch defenders of Christianity. But of one thing I am sure: I am sure that I fought not only for what I earnestly believed to be right but for the truest kind of religious freedom intended by the First Amendment, the complete separation of church and state.*

As long as the public school is used to recruit the child or to segregate the children according to religion or to use the truancy power of the public schools to make them go to religions classes, I'm against it.

Note: Varied sources were examined for the bios of and quotes from the chosen luminaries. However, special appreciation goes out to the Freedom From Religion Foundation's (FFRF) *Freethought of the Day* feature, particularly to Anne Laurie Gaylor, Bill Dunn and Sabrina Gaylor.

A Conversation With God

In the Beginning

Don and Grant were chatting on Skype one evening discussing the meaning of life, the origins of the universe and all things WO when God joined their conversation. He wasn't invited but he imposed his omnipresence, as Gods are want to do.

God: I was listening to your WO conversation and was intrigued. I have been around for a long time but have never heard such a discussion before. I have always known life has no meaning and the universe spontaneously erupted out of dark matter but what are WOs?

Don: WOs are so powerful they help people accomplish health goals, such as getting fit and becoming more energetic and cheerful, even when tired, stressed, desperate or depressed.

Grant: WOs are at the center of all good feelings. They are blocked or enhanced by the way we see the world, where we live, with whom we live, the conversations we have and how we interpret those conversations.

Don: We believe that hanging out with healthy, happy individuals will make anyone healthy and happy, over time. What's more, it will increase their WO count exponentially, while they sit around waiting to die, and it sure beats hanging out with depressing religious types.

God: I agree about the religious types, they really are one big stuff-up. But let's be clear about one thing; they're not my doing.

Grant: So you never asked some guy called Abraham to start a religion?

God: I do remember a guy named Abraham that I chatted with a few thousand years back but I never asked him to start a religion. I think I said, "You're only going to be here for a short time so why not religiously seek out fun wherever you can find it?" I guess he missed the point.

Don: You're not kidding. He spawned three disasters.

Grant: But, your omnipotence, don't you have the power to see everything in the Universe as it happens? Why didn't you stop him once he got going?

God: Hey, lay off the omnipotence bit. I'm just plain God, that's all. As to putting the brakes on that idiot Abraham, what do you expect of me? I don't have any superpowers?

Don: That's pretty much the story they're peddling down here.

God: Well, they would be stupid. I can benevolently tap into a computer chat or listen in like the NSA or Chinese military but I'm not supernatural or anything. I'm long-lived, I'll give you that, and I'm pretty good at seeing the big picture but that's about my limit. I'm just trying to live a WO-filled life myself but, when I look around, all I see are Muslims, Jews and Christians destroying everything they touch. It's awful.

Grant: Well, can't you break in and have a chat with the pope, the bishops, the cardinals, the imams, rabbis, monks, televangelists and all the rest who are purporting to represent you?

God: I could, sure, but why waste my time? They don't take me any more seriously than you two do. Besides, they're so bloody pompous and dogmatic. I don't think I could have a rational conversation with any of them. They don't have your rational, exuberant, athletic and liberty-based approach to life, so they are very hard work.

Don: So, let me see if we understand your point. You like REAL wellness and now what? You want us to be messengers, prophets, apostles or some kind of disciples for WO?

God: Whoa. Let's not get carried away. I didn't break into this little chat to aggrandize, elevate, levitate or transubstantiate you two. I just said you're on the right track. Don't go all Abraham on me. But, speaking of prophets and messengers, the best things going on when the holy books were written were largely ignored.

Grant: What do you mean?

God: Well, way too much attention has been given to self-proclaimed prophets and too little to the Romans who were building roads, digging aqueducts and laying sewer lines. These initiatives enhanced quality of life. They boosted public health, provided fresh water and warded off disease. They made life easier but who gets all the press? The guy spreading false hope, promising pie in the sky, endless WOs in a non-existent afterlife.

Don: Makes me think of Eric Idle on a cross in *The Life of Brian*, singing about always looking on the bright side of life.

God: God, I love that song. Especially the ending:

> *I mean, what have you got to lose?*
> *You know, you come from nothing.*
> *You're going back to nothing.*
> *What have you lost? Nothing.*

Grant: God, now you're here I have so many questions about animals and plants, purposes for one life form or another, about the persistence of evil, about meaning, about eternity and how that all works, about other worlds, about love ...

Don: Yeah, and whether life extension is possible and ...

Grant: God?

Don: God, are you there?

Don: I think he's gone.

Grant: Why did you have to bring up life extension?

Don: Well, hell, you asked about eternity, for god's sake.

Grant: I think we lost him.

Don: I'm not sure we ever had him.

To be continued.......

www.ingramcontent.com/pod-product-compliance
Lightning Source LLC
Chambersburg PA
CBHW050400290526
45786CB00003B/1059